NAKED FITNESS I

REVEALING THE "BARE" TRUTH ABOUT YOUR HEALTH & FITNESS

KEVIN DURIO

ISBN: 978-1-4834-7702-2 (sc)
ISBN: 978-1-4834-7701-5 (e)

Lulu Publishing Services rev. date: 11/28/2017

Contents

Introduction

What is fitness? When the majority of people talk about fitness, the first thing that comes to mind is losing some fat, getting lean and "cut", body building, getting into a certain pair of jeans or bathing suit, eating healthy, exercise, sweating, sets and reps, and in general being physically active and looking like your "fit" friend or that magazine cover. Fitness IS all of that of course, and … it's totally achievable by EVERYONE who really wants it. Yeah, we all know that, right?? Well, why then are there still so many unfit and unhealthy people out there?? Guys and gals … we're headed down a road where this country has one third of its population near or at the obese level! We gotta do something fast! Families from other countries, whom have never had an overweight or obesity issue in their family, come to America and within one generation have exactly that. What does that tell you?

Physical fitness can best be described as a planned and consistent path of repeated exercises and nutritional practices in an effort to gain muscular and cardiovascular strength, as part of a physically healthy foundation for living. So it is with the other fitness foundations of your life; they too will take planned and consistent actions to make them a part of *your* healthy life, leading you to a balanced and fit lifestyle. Just as a house needs solid ground to add stability and strength for its longevity, these four foundations are the key to a healthy, complete and more balanced way of living.

In this book series, I'll outline these four foundations as the ground floor of Naked Fitness. The four foundations are basic to every one of us. They fit every person and every lifestyle and every income. After reading this series you'll be able to give a more comprehensive and realistic answer to the question; what is fitness?

The four foundations of Naked Fitness that are extremely important if one is to be "totally fit" are:

- Physical fitness
- Spiritual fitness
- Financial fitness
- Mental fitness

Not necessarily in that order, but now you know where we're headed! Each one of these foundations is absolutely fundamental to everyone on the planet. With these foundations in place, a balanced, complete and full life is yours for the living, and life *IS* for living and living means learning and learning means growth ... and growth rocks! I've heard it said, the PURPOSE of life is to live a life of purpose. I truly believe we all have a "job" to do while on this planet. I believe we all have talents and skills for that job ... we just have to be brave enough and ask enough questions to find the right avenues to express those skills. I believe these four foundations are a great beginning to that journey.

Why Naked Fitness? There is so much junk science and junk equipment out there right now, all trying to convince you that this or that product is the only thing you need to use, or this or that new "berry" is the best food on the planet to eat and you're not at the top of your game if you're not using that piece of equipment or eating that berry ... and it's mostly junk information!! My goal is twofold; **FIRST**, I don't want to promote a certain way to live other than to present ideas that you can choose to incorporate into your life as you see fit, no pun intended, but if something in the fitness section catches your attention and you feel it's valuable to you, then go with it and incorporate it. If something catches your attention in the faith section, then do your own homework to see if it blends with your current belief system. If a thought hits you in the financial section, then I encourage you to talk with your family and your accountant to make the appropriate changes for the better, and then repeat the same with the other chapters.

SECOND, I do want to promote a "back to basics" strategy that you can follow for the rest of your life. If you're new to exercise, then this will be a solid base to work from. If you're an experienced exerciser, then this might be the point where you remember how it all started and want to get back to something sustainable long term. This also applies to other foundations ... "back to basics" is your new mantra. Bruce Lee said it best; "It's not about the increase, it's about the daily decrease, hack away at the unessential." Now, he was mostly talking about the martial arts, but this idea works in any area of life.

There are countless ridiculous diets as well as an endless supply of stupid fitness myths floating around; it's no wonder everyone is confused and feels mislead so easily. This book will not be some "high-browed", technically laid out, fancy worded addition to all that junk, and it won't be a "dummy" book that pretends to be easy to understand and could still be a college level semester of technical facts and calculations. It's setup as a step-by-small-step handbook to get you to your workout faster and with more CLEAR information about what to do and how to do it than ever before. It is my strong belief that you really do know the basics of how to be fit, you've just been turned around and thrown all over the place with fancy acronyms and new jumbled up words that make it sound like it's all brand new stuff when it isn't. All I want to do is dispel as many of those fitness and diet myths and stupid junk that the fitness industry perpetuates to make you spend money to do and buy crap you DO NOT NEED, as I can!! I'm not angry at my profession, just really REALLY tired of all the "junk science" in the fitness world. Every industry has its over-the-top stupid side, but for some reason the fitness industry has a LOT more stupid stuff in it. Probably because it's as easy to get to as walking into any gym and seeing people repeating the dumb stuff they see online. Even today, a guy or a gal, with no formal education in health and fitness, and all too often, with no real experience, can go and take a personal training certification course over a week or even worse, just a weekend and then go to work at a gym or start home training and tell YOU how to be fit. Ummm ...

So you lost your way down the fitness path or just never found the trailhead, no worries, I'm going to help you. Your body was made to be fit ... you just gotta wake it up by getting started. This book will help serve as a solid guide to giving you that jumpstart and maintaining a fit lifestyle. This first volume won't be a fitness "manual" outlining individual workouts for this type of person or that type of blood or that type shape, blah blah blah ... but it will be a detailed guide to help you sort through a lot of the junk information that is ridiculously prevalent in the fitness industry, putting you in a greater position to make better choices and start better habits for physical health. It's also my goal to give you as much help as I can to motivate you to get your butt moving. So, I've also included a web address just in case you have any questions and want to bounce your fitness thoughts off me. If you're already lean, healthy and have a regular fitness program that you've committed to, then you're doing the fitness component correctly, keep up the good work and look at the following information as a solid review and maybe you'll find a new idea or two. If you're not engaged in regular exercise, then read on and get started.

The best suggestion I have on how to use this book is to read each chapter a couple of times to let the message sink in. Within each chapter I've put websites, references and key points to help you find more information on that particular subject if you chose to follow up. With this in mind, here are a few more thoughts to help guide you through the four foundations to Naked Fitness.

How well do you think a plant would grow if you just randomly threw some seeds onto the sidewalk? Even with perfect sunlight and some water, it wouldn't grow without soil, right? So it is with humans. It's certainly not enough to have great *physical* health or great *financial* health alone and so on. You must also have the other basic elements to live a balanced life. Think for a second, and be honest with yourself, what if you had the money of a billionaire but markedly poor health with no ability to enjoy any real measure of life? How miserable might it be to have all that money *and* the health to enjoy spending it, but have no friends or family? Sure you could "buy" some friends, but you and I both know how hollow that would be. Now, what if I offered you one million dollars cash for just one of your arms or one of your legs? Or would you take five million dollars and let me remove either both arms or both legs? How much would you take to let me remove your sight? Is 10 million dollars enough for me to take away your mental health? What if you have great health, close family and friends, a high IQ as well as common sense, your soul is in check with your faith, but for whatever reason, you don't have a dime to your name and depend on others for every other basic need? I'm sure you can see where I'm going with these questions. When you stop and think about these four foundations to a balanced life, you might agree that we need all of them to stand on our own; no short-cuts. The four foundations to Naked Fitness *are* the solid ground on which you can build a strong house; one that can weather any storm. As you've seen, to be rid of just one of these four foundations would without a doubt weaken the base your house sits on and it would certainly crack if not crumble.

Look what happened in 2009 - the investment scams that came to light - a very wounded Wall Street - all the bailouts - a down economy with people losing their jobs, savings and retirement funds. It put real strains on families, and that was only one of the foundations. I'm positive many people also experienced losses in the other foundations as well. The events certainly stressed people out (mental), that in turn effects the body (physical), a lot of folks questioned some of their life choices and why this was happening to them (spiritual) ... all the foundations were affected by the one (financial).

We, as a nation, have experienced hard times in the past, and we'll have more in the future. This book in no way professes to be a disaster-proof plan but it certainly won't hurt you to have strong foundations as it is outlined in the following pages. You could possibly go a long way with one of the foundations out of step with the others, but it'll catch-up with you eventually. The stress and strain on the other foundations to maintain balance will have an impact in your life, even more so if you're not prepared and do not have a strong and solid base. I'm not claiming to have all the answers for everyone in every situation, but if what you read here makes sense to you, then by all means feel free to follow along and use whatever you find helpful.

Keep in mind that you need to do your own homework and get your questions answered from specialists you trust in the areas presented. I'm happy to give you guidelines and point you in the right direction, but don't just go off and try something out of this series without looking into it yourself. You'll see all through these books where I say: do your homework ... or ... look it up for yourself and consult whomever ... that's also why I put bullet reminders and the references at the end of every chapter, so they're handy and fresh in your head. You need to be smart and use the references to protect yourself from the stupidity being thrown around out in the fitness world today.

I wrote this book to share with you my belief that these four foundations are the pathway to a really healthy and more complete life. It's my wish that you will enjoy reading it and find something valuable you can use as well. IF you are ready to sort through all the unnecessary crap out of a really simple subject, then read on!!!

Have fun and good reading ... and good living!

PHYSICAL FITNESS
(the "bare" essentials)

Let's start with a very basic definition and explanation of "physical fitness". Physical fitness can best be described as a planned and consistent program of repeated exercises and practices in an effort to gain muscular and cardiovascular strength, as well as good nutritional habits ... pretty simple, right? Well... actually, it is really simple to have and <u>maintain</u> good health and fitness ... it's the "getting" there that most people have a really hard time with and don't like. I mean, you gotta **want** to get lean and fit and the only way to get there is to be disciplined enough to stick to your goals like super glue. You'll want to give up – almost every workout, you'll want to sleep in – almost every morning, you'll want to skip your afternoon / evening workout to go get a beer or dinner with friends, you'll want to binge on your favorite junk food from time to time ... you're going to be tempted to quit, but you have to get through all of that to reach your goal, and believe me ... it will be worth it! That's the hard part though, you're not alone. EVERYBODY wants the end result ... but ONLY the ones that *really* want it, and stick it out to the end, make it to the end.

Let me put this thought in your head; our bodies are **NOT** "sedentary" vehicles; they are made to move and to move well and smooth for a long time. WE jack them up with bad food, a lack of physical activity, drugs (not necessarily illegal either) and alcohol, and the amazing thing is ... they keep working!!! That right there is why most people think "see, I'm ok, I don't need to exercise, I can still do ...", maybe you can "still do" whatever ... but you could most certainly do it better AND do more of it if you were exercising & eating cleaner food.

Now, here's another "truth" that should take away some anxiety about your path to health and fitness; you **<u>DO NOT</u>** have to be a triathlete or marathon runner or fitness instructor or live in a gym for hours at a time or be a competitive "bodybuilder" or be a devotee to any specialized TV fitness program to be active and considered fit and healthy. Now, if being one of those things is something you really want to be, then go for it, but do not let anyone lead you to believe that that's the only way to be fit. Same thing goes for all the "fad fitness" programs out there. You'd think they were a new religion the way their members talk about the program and look down at everyone that **ISN'T** doing that particular program – what a bunch of knuckleheads! The vast majority of these types of programs are really okay ... in the short term, but they are unsustainable in the long run, and a lot of people that get in thinking they'll be fit in no time, will hurt themselves trying to push to crazy levels too quickly!

Keep this mind ... YOU CAN'T **CRAM** YOUR FITNESS!!! You never could and you never will. Proper fitness is an on-going, daily / weekly / monthly / yearly thing. Fitness is not an "event", fitness is a lifestyle. The "event" is the event; fitness just lets you do that event better. Fitness is not something you do to get ready for "that" event 4 to 6 to 8 weeks away, like a wedding or vacation or bikini pool time. True fitness IS a lifestyle that you live all year long so you don't have to get ready for something ... you already are ready for it!! Having said that, obviously there is "specific" training you can & should do to get ready for a special run or other specific competition ... whatever it is, but you should ALREADY have a solid base of fitness year 'round and not cramming it in and hoping to just make it through. 'Makes sense, right? When you decide to start any fitness program or join a class at the gym, just start slow and steady and do it correctly from the start and you'll go a long way to having fun with it AND preventing injury.

Unfortunately, steroid use among the youth is still going on strong as ever and it's really sad! We had a young man at a gym I was working out of that was obviously taking steroids. The fact that even a handful of members noticed how he ballooned up just over a summer, made it important enough for me to approach him. I confronted him about it and mentioned how he's headed down a bad path ... he obviously denied it and even said that he appreciated me "thinking" that he was doing it because it meant that he was working hard! Can you believe that stupidity? Like I couldn't see and tell that he was "juicing", I mean, that's my job to know this stuff. That's like asking a cop; "how can you tell I'm breaking a law"? Unfortunately, it's not just the guys getting into all that. I see girls that want to get stronger and, actually bigger, and think that taking the extra supplements will help them – sure it will, but only in the short term and only with consequences. Taking growth hormone (unless prescribed by a doctor for a legitimate illness) or the "amped up" products out on the market to get healthier is stupid beyond belief.

I really hate to do this because deep down I honestly do respect the dedication of these athletes and what it takes to compete, but I'm not making it up; take competitive "bodybuilding" as it's practiced today. It's not the healthiest thing you can do for your body. They're taking certain drugs / supplements to grow their muscles faster, taking others to shred or "cut" (simply meaning to lose fat and make the skin-to-muscle connection as small or thin as possible so you can see their muscles better), taking more to get "amped" for the workout and then that night taking something else to sleep. They fatten up in the off season and then put their body through stages of calorie deprivation on the road to the competition, so you can see how "cut" they get. All of that just to have a "look" goes against all health habits and findings of proper body management, its crazy unhealthy for you on several levels. The men and women that do this kind of body building are athletes for sure, but this kind of training is not for the average Joe or Jill. Having said all of that, "natural body builders" don't have all the answers either; they're just not taking all the extra supplements. They have frequent drug tests and they stick to all-natural foods and combinations of natural supplements. This is still NOT the answer to ALL fitness questions, but it is a better option by far.

This is not just a "body builder" issue; on-again / off-again periods hit ALL athletes at some point. Every single athlete at every level and in every sport has experienced this at one time in their careers. Just be aware that it can and most likely will get you as well. Once you notice a "slide" in that direction, make corrections, taper your training, keep moving and do your best not to fall into bad habits that will totally derail what you're doing. A slip now and then is a slip now and then, it happens … just keep it short and to a minimum.

Ok, you don't have to be a high level athlete or competitive bodybuilder to experience an on again / off again weight loss plan. Even if you try a different diet plan every year, you're going to experience the on again / off again of changing diets. While the actual effects of the on again / off again isn't "bad" for you like many want to think it is, it is still crazy flawed as a sustainable healthy plan for body weight management. Let's look at this "yo-yo" process and what it does to you. *(1)*

- First; you make a decision to lose weight – whether you do it with an existing plan or try something on your own, here is where you start. You begin your exercises and eating cleanly; you might even join a gym and try some classes or hire a trainer. You're excited to get going.
- Next; you reach a few quick goals and make a few visible changes. Your friends notice and encourage you and now you're really off and running.
- Now comes the hard part; maintaining ... keeping up the pace you've set to get to this point. You feel you're having to work harder to see results, and the results you saw happen quickly in the beginning are now few and far between if at all. This could be for several reasons; overtraining to make gains, not resting properly, or just the basics of you losing weight and it becoming much harder to lose those few last pounds. That's called hitting a "plateau."
- The next thing that happens, all too often, is when someone hits a plateau, they lose motivation; the weight isn't coming off like it used to, the workouts are losing their excitement, one of your friends has already quit his / her program and now they're slacking a bit and now you're doubting your own efforts. You begin to indulge again in a few of your favorite junk foods and lazy behavior ... that's called a "slip-up."
- Finally; you fall off your program completely and stop going to the gym, stop making better choices when you go out to eat or when you choose a snack, you gain a few pounds back and

then a few more, you're not exercising so you watch TV more and sit around more and so on.

- Then one day you get the bug again and you start over and this time you think you have a better plan, so you set your weight loss goals again, rejoin your gym, notify your friends ... and now you reach for one of those fad-fitness and fad-diet plans to do it "right," or you might go to your local vitamin store and get "supplements" to help with your new plan (keep in mind, the vast majority of the supplements in any vitamin store or even your local grocery store, or NOT regulated or approved by FDA. Anyone can invent a mixture; call it a proprietary blend and you won't know what's in or not in it.) You're hoping it'll work this time, and it honestly just might, but the numbers are not in your favor so, the process repeats itself, except this time the crash is worse because now you've introduced these "supplements" and one of those fad-fitness programs. You get crazy excited and you're working hard and then it happens ... you get hurt trying to make up for the time you lost sitting on your butt watching TV. Now you have to take time off to care for that injury and heal. Take the time THIS time to re-evaluate and make a better, more sustainable plan for your health and fitness.

I tell my clients all the time that everyone is either "fit", "deconditioned" or "unfit". What's the difference you might ask? Here is how I define these;

FIT is exactly that – you workout on a regular basis and you watch what you eat the majority of the time. You're active and live a healthy lifestyle. You use the stairs more than you don't and you reach for sweets only as an occasional treat. Your weight and body fat are in check and in a healthy range. You get your health checkups each year. You're doing fine.

DECONDITIONED means - you were fit at one time, maybe months ago or even years ago, but you were fit and exercising and then something happened. Maybe you had an injury, or had a child or had a prolonged illness, job loss or job change that jacked up your schedule or even simply ... you changed or lost your goal. For whatever reason, you got off track. You CAN get your fitness back; you're just temporarily ... deconditioned. Your body was fit and knew what that felt like. It wants to feel that way again!

UNFIT is the ugliest one – you haven't voluntarily put out one drop of sweat in your life. The last time you did any exercise was during your early childhood in PE class or at recess, and you hated it. God bless you, for some reason you've now picked up this book and I do hope and pray something speaks to you to continue on to good health. Y'all are an exciting group to train and play with because you guys and gals will see, feel & reap the greatest benefits when the benefits start to show. Not to mention the emotional boost you'll get from seeing your body, your mood, your confidence ... all of that and so much more will change in a very positive way!

We have all sorts of current technologies that make a good bit of our work a lot less physical, so a few (far too few) of us make time for our health by being active. The rest of us don't. **STOP** looking at exercise as a luxury thing. Health and fitness is not for any ONE class or group of people, it **IS** for **everyone**. If you have a body, you need to move it and exercise it ... PERIOD! If you eat, have bones and muscles and move around during the day ... you have **NO** excuse to be unfit. There is **NO** excuse to not do **some** body movement, **some** kind of play, **some** light activity and then, **some** planned exercise. I work in a gym most of the time and love being a trainer and love my job in general, but you do not have to go to a gym to be fit and healthy. You already own the greatest piece of fitness equipment known to man ... your body!! Having said that, in a later chapter I go into the hows and whys of joining a gym if that's what you want to do.

So, the take home message of this chapter is to move your body most days of the week with one solid day of rest. In rest is where you repair, rebuild and recharge from all the stuff you put your body through in the past week. Just don't rest too much!!!

(1) http://www.medicinenet.com/script/main/art.
asp?articlekey=21745

The WRAP:

- Your body is not a sedentary vehicle
- You do not have to be a fitness pro or some extreme athlete to be considered fit and healthy
- You CAN'T cram your fitness
- You're either FIT or DECONDITIONED or UNFIT ... aim to be "fit"
- There is NO excuse to be "unfit"
- You don't have to join a gym to be fit and healthy
- Find ANY reason to move and exercise ... it WILL pay off for you

BENEFITS OF EXERCISE

(the "bare" minimum)

"The benefits of being fit are many; there are **NO** benefits to being unfit." I love the simplicity and truth of this quote. Being healthy is worth more than all the gold in the world, being unfit ... is worth absolutely nothing!!! I mean, no amount of money can buy you real health and fitness ... maybe a fancy scooter or walker with all kinds of bells and whistles, but that's it. No need to go on about it ... we all KNOW that it's better to be healthy and fit than not. Here's a short list of the most notable benefits to being fit and exercising regularly.

BENEFITS OF A STRUCTURED EXERCISE PROGRAM

The positives of exercise are well documented *(1)*, but here are some explanations of just a few of them. Like I said in the beginning, this book hits the very basics of this subject because real fitness isn't all that complicated, it is a lot of common sense though. If you're not making money with your fitness, as in a paid athlete, or you're not an Olympian ... then fitness should be really simple ... basic. Ok, enough of that, here we go.

- **Lowers your blood pressure** – in general terms, the more fit and clean your cardiovascular system is (heart and respiratory system/lungs with all its attachments and arteries and vessels), the easier it is for the heart to move blood and nutrients around your body. If you think of the heart as a mechanical pump, it will obviously run better with good maintenance and running CLEAN fluids through it as well as having open and clear hoses in the system. So it is with the heart – keeping it strong and running clean blood and good nutrients through it helps it run smoother and better thus lowering the pressure (your blood pressure) in the hoses – your arteries and vessels – not to mention the cleaner the blood the less cholesterol and plaque. Some excellent examples of cardio exercise; walking, jogging, biking, rowing, swimming ... keep in mind, you DO NOT have to be breaking records with any of these exercises to get a benefit, just get up and move. *(1)*

- **Decreases stress & improves your mood -** exercise decreases stress by burning excess energy and releasing hormones and neurotransmitters as well as the much touted endorphins that enable the mind and body to cope with inside and outside stressors. Not to mention, when you do cardio or weight training exercises you are in effect tightening and loosening your entire body. It's like getting a massage that relaxes as well as strengthens muscle. Exercise has been described as meditation in motion, by taking your mind off the daily junk and worries of the day and relieving both mind and body of stress. Even a little stress releases cortisol – a fat storing/producing hormone. Exercise will burn off any excess cortisol in the system so as not to be stored. Stress also releases adrenaline – produced in the adrenal glands that prepare the body for fight or flight. Once you've slowed or stopped the stressor, levels of cortisol and adrenaline return to normal. Too much or on-going stress produces what's called *chronic stress* which keeps these hormones and chemicals in the system which can and does do damage to the body and certain organs. Exercise most definitely helps keep these hormones in check. *(1)*
- **Gives you energy –** the exercise energy paradox says; the more energy you expend as in exercise, the more you have to spend. Now don't go splitting hairs, we all know you can overdo it by overtraining, and of course you won't have any extra energy - but for the sake of argument, by being engaged in regular exercise you actually energize the body by keeping it ready and primed for even more activity. The bodies we have today are meant to be moved and moved a lot. If you want more "energy" in your day ... use some energy and get to exercising. *(1)*

- **Boosts your immune system** – exercise teaches the body to take on physical stress and that in turn boosts the body's ability to fight off attacks to the immune system. That's the simple explanation, here's a little more; moderate exercise has been linked to a positive immune system response and a temporary boost in the production of macrophages (large phagocytes that engulf and digests debris and invading microorganisms). Another benefit is that during exercise, certain immune cells similar to macrophages are being distributed throughout the body and are able to kill additional bacteria and viruses. After exercise ends, the immune system generally returns to normal within a few hours, but consistent and regular exercise seems to make these changes more long lasting. Studies show that even recreational and moderate exercisers report fewer colds and sickness once they began a regular exercise program. *(1)(2)*
- **Maintains and/or strengthens bone mass** – bone is alive like any other part of your body, just like the muscles that are attached to it. Once you put a stress on the muscle and increase its "tension", as in exercise, that translates to tension on the bone through the tendons, thereby stimulating the bone to grow stronger by creating new bone cells, to hold the new stress. That's a simple way to say that weight / strength training can and does slow, didn't say STOP, bone degeneration, if caught in time. Current studies *(3)(4)* have shown a very positive connection to moderate weight training and a fairly dramatic slowing of osteoporosis signs and symptoms, even in the elderly population of 70+ years of age.
- **Speeds up your metabolism and burns fat** – when you exercise you increase the speed at which your body burns "fuel", i.e., carbohydrates and fat. Ever notice when you get into exercising regularly how hungry you are almost all the time? That's because lean muscle, like you get when your

muscles are toned and tight, burns calories even at rest. That means more fat burned even when you're not exactly exercising at that very moment - cool uh!? *(1)*

- **Helps you sleep better –** simply put, when you exercise you use up energy, a lot of it! Therefore it makes sense that you'd have to rest to re-energize, re-pair and re-build. When you workout, you are in effect tearing down your muscle and muscle needs rest to fix itself and grow to meet the demands you're putting on it. You'll get the bulk of your rest when you sleep, and sleep you will if you're exercising on a regular basis. In a nut-shell, rest is just as important to good health as the exercise itself. YOU DO NOT NEED TO WORKOUT 7 DAYS A WEEK TO GET A BENEFIT. In fact you'll be going backward in a hurry if you workout like that, that's called "overtraining" and too many of you, especially if you're in one of those "fad fitness" programs, are doing just that. Even Olympic athletes rest as part of their training regimen. If it's good enough for them ... it's definitely good enough for us!!! Stop trying to keep up with that loud mouthed knucklehead in the gym that "thinks" he's an Olympian. More than likely he's downing fake energy in the form of "amped up" drinks and thermogenic pills just to get through the workout. Believe me; he's not "healthier" than you. Not exercising, not eating clean, eating late, alcohol, drugs and too much caffeine all contribute to not sleeping well and that means low energy levels. So what do most of us do to boost our energy? We intake extra loads of caffeine and those stupid energy drinks and energy "pills". Then we rest far too much when we really do run out of energy. When we wake up we're tired and groggy and need to get going again so ... we take an energy pill or drink and ... start the whole mess over again. It's a bad cycle that far too many of us are in right at this very moment thinking we're getting fit. We're not. Rest is where you repair, rebuild & recharge.

You CANNOT get bigger or stronger or faster or even leaner without proper rest. Your body needs rest to get and do all the above. There is no way around it. Oh sure, you can get by for a little while, but if health and fitness really is your goal, you gotta have rest in your program. Okay then, what is proper rest?? Take one whole day each week & do **NO** exercise at all, then take another day each week and do "active rest" which essentially is "playing" and not a structured workout. Go for a walk, play with the kids, ride your bike, stretch ... just be active and NOT "working out". That still leaves you with 5 days of the week for working out – make the most of those 5 days and earn your rest days! *(1)*

- **Better sex –** ohhh yeah, that's right, I said better sex. All kinds of science "bare" this out - pun intended. The more fit you are, the more physical you can be. The body works better when it's strong and lean AND ... you'll last longer – guy or girl – with a strong cardiovascular system getting blood flow to all the important parts of the body for better sex. Because exercise burns fat as well, having less body fat is an extra bonus ... especially when you're *naked* in front of someone ... 'just saying, "wink"!

Ok, that should've answered a few of your questions about the benefits of exercise. Now, let's talk about a few other "basics" you should be aware of like ... your weight, your body fat % and the BMI.

(1) http://www.mayoclinic.org/healthy-lifestyle/fitness/ in-depth/exercise/art-20048389
(2) http://www.webmd.com/cold-and-flu/cold-guide/ exercise-when-you-have-cold
(3) http://www.niams.nih.gov/Health_Info/Bone/Bone_Health/ Exercise/default.asp
(4) http://www.mayoclinic.org/diseases-conditions/ osteoporosis/in-depth/osteoporosis/ART-20044989

The WRAP:

- Lower blood pressure
- Decreases stress & improves your mood
- Gives you energy
- Boosts your immune system
- Maintains and strengthens bone mass
- Speeds up metabolism and burns fat
- Helps you sleep more soundly
- Better sex

BODY WEIGHT BASICS

(the "naked" truth)

STOP saying you want to lose weight! If you're thinking that you want to "just lose some weight" then ... cut something off!! That's loosing weight. What you really want to have happen is to lose "inches". The correct thinking of losing weight is to lose inches and accept the fact that your weight may not go down – it might even go up a bit - but if you're losing "inches" and your clothes are fitting better or you're having to punch a new hole in your belt to tighten it up ... then you're doing it the right way. The other thing about "just losing some weight" is ... you want to have a specific goal with the weight you have in mind to lose. "Just losing some weight" won't get you to the first pound. You really want to be as specific as possible and also take advantage of using an end-date as well. An "end date" is just that, a date that you want to reach your goal. It really does help!

To help you get comfortable with the idea that your weight might go up a bit, keep this in mind; lean muscle, the kind you get from regular exercise, is heavier than fat. That's science, that's a fact, that won't change. Your arm or leg or belly ... whatever is your main concern ... doesn't have to get "bigger" to be strong and lean and heavier than before, in fact just the opposite is more true than not. When you first start working out, especially with weights or specific strength training, your muscle will first "feel" tight and maybe a bit sore because you are doing something with it that it hasn't ever done or maybe not in a long time. The muscle tightens up and gets denser because you're creating more muscle cells to handle the load you're putting on it. It doesn't just "grow" and get huge from the first or second or tenth workout ... it takes more and it takes fueling (eating) a certain way and in certain amounts to make muscles really GROW, oh yeah ... not to mention a certain amount of genetics as well. Your muscles will feel bigger from the first workout because you're putting blood and nutrients and oxygen in them and they'll **feel** puffed up. They might even look puffed up for a bit, but that's only temporary. That's the "pump" you hear guys and gals talking about. That feeling will settle down a bit after the workout and you'll lose that "pumped" look as well after a bit, but be assured, new muscle cells *are* beginning to grow from the first workout.

The other thing about your weight is that, it'll fluctuate as much as one to six pounds a day, just get that in your head & get over it. Quit freaking out about weighing every day. All you're doing is putting more stress on yourself for thinking and worrying about how much you weigh. Think of your fluctuating weight like this; you weigh more after lunch than you did before, you'll weigh less after you go potty than before. You weigh less and less as you burn food / fuel as you're moving around during the day and exercising. Weighing only tells you how much *all* of YOU weigh at that moment ... all the skin, muscle, blood, bone, poo, pee, any food in the colon, arms and legs and head ... your scale at the house and at your gym, doesn't break it down for you ... you just weigh what you weigh. You can extrapolate fat loss a number of ways as we'll explore in this chapter, but my point is to not obsess over or about your weight without understanding the basics.

And while we're on the subject of weighing ...don't bother with those home or gym scales that tell you your body fat as well. Most of these scales use what's called bio-impedance *(1),* Bioelectrical impedance measures the resistance of different body tissues through the flow of a small and harmless electrical signal through the bottom of your feet as you stand on the metal pads or through the palm of your hands if it's a hand-held model. It calculates your body fat percentage as the current flows more easily through the parts of the body that are composed mostly of water (such as blood, urine and muscle) than it does through bone, fat or air. It is possible to predict how much body fat a person has by combining the bioelectric impedance measure with other factors such as height, weight, gender, fitness level and age. It's certainly not exact, but it will get you in the ballpark. It also takes into consideration how hydrated you are or aren't – that'll effect your numbers as well. A bio-impedance scale can be off by as much as four to seven points either way, up or down. That simply means if you were actually

20% body fat, it'll tell you that you're either 13-16% (not a bad fat %, but still very off) or 24-27%. That's a BIG difference when you're trying to track your progress. Some of them even have a button you can push and change the setting to something like "athlete" and that's supposed to "fine tune" your fat percentage ... but you did NOTHING but push a button. Remember, this works by sending an electric current through your body – the same body you used just a few seconds before – but now that you've pushed that button ... it gives you a completely different number??? There's something wrong with that. Remember also, this method takes into consideration your level of hydration and if you're not a water drinker – as I know this to be the case for a lot of you out there - your results can vary wildly, couple that with what we said above about it being off four to seven % to start with and that makes this method of fat determination mostly inaccurate. You can get a little better reading with more sophisticated devices that send the electric signal through both your hands AND your feet -- increasing the accuracy.

Also, don't be confused that "looking" fit means that you are. "Skinny" doesn't necessarily mean you're fit nor have lean muscle. There's a case to be made that being "skinny" actually leads to poor bone health, it's called Osteoporosis. In a nut shell, when you put stress on a muscle, such as in weight or strength training or even physical labor, that "stress" puts tension on the bones through the muscles and tendons and that makes the bones produce more bone cells (osteocytes) to strengthen the bone to handle the stress, making the bones stronger. So my point is; being "skinny" doesn't necessarily translate to having strong, lean muscle or real muscle mass. Remember, exercise is only one part of an osteoporosis prevention or treatment program. A diet rich in calcium and vitamin D and exercise helps strengthen bones at any age.

Having said that, please keep in mind that proper exercise and diet may not be enough to stop bone loss caused by medical conditions, menopause, or lifestyle choices such as tobacco use and excessive alcohol consumption. It's really important to visit with your doctor about your bone health. Guys, don't think for a second that osteoporosis is a "ladies" disease, osteoporosis is a "bone" disease, so if you have bones ... you're susceptible. Ask your family physician if you could be a candidate for a bone mineral density test. If you are diagnosed with low bone mass, see what your doctor recommends to stave off the disease and help keep your bones strong. He / she should recommend some form of weight bearing exercise as well as medical supplementation.

Ken Cooper of The Cooper Clinic in Dallas, Texas, proved that you can get stronger at almost ANY age in almost ANY condition. You just have to want to. The best exercise for your bones is the weight-bearing kind, which forces you to work against gravity. Some examples of weight-bearing exercises include weight / strength training, walking, hiking, jogging, climbing stairs, tennis, and dancing. Examples of exercises that are not weight-bearing include swimming and bicycling. Although these activities help build and maintain strong muscles and have **excellent** cardiovascular benefits, they are not the best way to exercise your bones. Be honest about your health and start working out to be healthy and fit, not just "pretty". Pretty can easily be lipstick on a pig. Skinny doesn't mean fit, but **FIT** is "pretty" and being **FIT** is really sexy.

MORE ABOUT YOUR BODY FAT

Here are a few more ways to check your body fat. We mentioned above about the bio-impedance weight scales and how they figure your body fat percentage. The other body fat method that you hear about and that's still out there – I have no idea why - is the Body Mass Index or BMI. The BMI is a measure of someone's weight in relation to their height. Everybody knows this stupid thing is crazy flawed and yet you still hear fitness people and a lot of physicians quote BMI numbers like its gospel ... **IT AINT!** In its definition is its flaw ... think about it, it's a measure of ones weight in relation to ones height ... okay then, if you're some "normal" height guy or gal, but really lean with a good muscle build (remember that muscle weighs more than fat), you might be carrying more weight than someone the same height ... in the BMI you could easily be classified as "overweight" to fat or obese.

Virtually every single "bodybuilder" is considered obese on the BMI scale just for the very reason that they are crazy lean with very dense muscle. They weigh a lot for their height. The chart will show them as obese and they're FAR from it. The BMI is a horrible way to track your "fatness" ... so don't use it.

This next one is much better than the others so far and if done correctly can get really close to the "gold standard" of water weighing (hydrostatic testing). This one is the three or seven fold pinch test. The one that most trainers use is the three pinch because it is fairly accurate and can be done quickly in a gym setting with little discomfort to you, the client. What happens is, the trainer will pinch you in three places (for guys it's the pectoral area, front of the belly and the front of the quad. For gals it's the back of the upper arm at the triceps, an angled spot at the iliac crest and the front of the quad) taking a measurement with the appropriate calipers that measures the thickness of the fat just under the surface of the skin, but NOT the muscle. Your trainer will then total up the numbers (which really are subject to the skill of the person measuring and the quality of the calipers) he / she gets from the three sites and look at a chart where the number and your age intersect and that's your body fat.

If done correctly, this test is very accurate and gets even better the more your trainer does it. I've been able to get within just a couple of points if not right on target against the water weighing (hydrostatic) test. I mentioned the seven fold pinch test, it's the same exact procedure and same sites plus four more that really fine tunes your body fat percentage number for more accurate tracking. Ask a trainer at your gym for this test.

The following are a few other methods that you can check your body fat with. Understand, just because I've mentioned it here doesn't mean you should use that particular option. I'm just making the point that there are many ways to get to the same conclusion. Some are very easy to get and are inexpensive and others are crazy out of range just to check your fat. The foundational theme of the Naked Fitness series is ... ***Do your own homework and be informed!!!***

DEXA Scan

DEXA or DXA stands for dual-emission X-ray absorptiometry. It's usually used for bone density testing, but it's also considered one of the most accurate ways to measure body fat. A DEXA scan is like getting a full-body X-ray, so it does deliver a small degree of radiation. You generally need a prescription and must visit a special clinic to have one done, and the whole work may cost hundreds or even thousands of dollars. For extremely overweight people, DEXA scans may be off by three to five percent.

HYDROSTATIC WEIGHING

Hydrostatic weighing involves submerging your body in water to determine your body density. Fat is less dense than muscle; thus, a person with a higher body fat will have a lower body density. You get into a dunk tank or pool, sit on the specially designed stool, and expel as much air as possible from your lungs. Many people find exhaling explosively to expel all their stored air challenging, so the results may be skewed slightly, up to two to three percent. You must visit a special facility to have the test performed; it can be really involved and maybe expensive, but it's more do-able than you might think.

AIR DISPLACEMENT PLETHYSMOGRAPHY

Air displacement Plethysmography, available commercially via a machine known as the BodPod, uses some of the same principles of hydrostatic weighing, but measures displaced air rather than water. As long ago as 1999, researchers declared air displacement Plethysmography as an accurate way to measure body composition. A later study published in a 2006 issue of Nutrition and Metabolism compared this method of measuring body composition against the DEXA scan and found that it measures changes in percentage of body fat similarly when someone is trying to lose weight. Availability of the method is limited, though, as machines are expensive. Professional sports teams and athletes are usually the primary users.

ALTERNATIVE ACCURATE METHODS

Some methods are exceptionally accurate, but not practical for most people. MRI and CT scans, for example, can distinguish between different types of tissue fairly readily, but they aren't usually necessary, or feasible, outside the clinical setting. They can even identify different types of fat - specifically visceral and subcutaneous fat. CT scans may deliver a high dose of radiation, though. The equipment used for both types of test is quite expensive and may not be able to hold people who are massively overweight.

THE IMPORTANCE (or unimportance) OF BODY FAT PERCENTAGE

Knowing what your body fat is when you start a workout program is honestly only somewhat important. It's only important to the point of making sure you're moving in the right direction, so checking it *periodically* over a period of time is quite appropriate, but you don't have to, and frankly shouldn't, check it daily or weekly or even monthly. The science *(2)* is fairly clear about body fat percentage and *some* metabolic disorders and diseases, so the take home message is, after you've gotten your baseline and know what your fat percentage is, and you've started your program & noticed a downward trend in your body fat ... **STOP** obsessing over it!!!! Now is when it's unimportant, now is when you pick out that pair of jeans you haven't been able to wear in awhile or that favorite little black dress or your favorite suit and tie / tux / evening gown, that you've worn in the past or your favorite pair of summer shorts or that special bathing suit / bikini ... put them out where you can see them every day and try them on every weekend until they do fit again. If you have them out and try them on often enough, I promise you, you'll fit in them sooner than you think.

Know your body fat percentage, understand what too much, and even too little, body fat can do to you. Women utilize body fat differently than men do and too little body fat can really screw up a woman's hormones and menstrual cycle – plus, I gotta tell ya, the majority of men want their wives, girlfriends and sisters to look "fit" and NOT like some walking skeleton. The same goes for women; they'd much rather their husbands, boyfriends and brothers not be skeletons either. Remember; one extreme is just as bad as the other. You'll want to know where you are and where you want to be, but after that, you gotta make it REAL by laying out some clothes that you really want to get back into. You don't care that a guy or gal your same age in some city across the country is in the same "body fat percentile" as you according to some medical chart ... who freakin cares ... you should care about getting back in those clothes you just laid out!

Women tend to carry the majority of their body fat on their upper legs and hips and arms ("wings"), and men tend to carry their body fat on the belly and upper body.

(1) http://www.topendsports.com/testing/tests/BI.htm
http://www.livestrong.com/article/436693-the-most-accurate-measurement-of-body-fat/
(2) http://www.mayoclinic.org/diseases-conditions/metabolic-syndrome/home/ovc-20197517

The WRAP:

- Losing "inches" and not weight is the correct and better way to view fat loss.
- Know your body fat to know where you're starting and where you're going.
- Your weight might actually go up – muscle weighs more than fat.
- Don't weigh every day or every week or even every month.
- Stop obsessing about weight.
- "Skinny" does **NOT** necessarily mean fit or healthy.
- Use a set of clothes as a real world measure of your progress.

NUTRITION BASICS

(and I mean "bare" BASIC)

First of all ... food **IS** fuel for the body, just like gas **IS** fuel for your car. I know that seems too simple, but seriously, I sincerely believe the vast majority of y'all know that food is important and you need to make smarter choices ... but you stop there and aren't thinking of food as actual "fuel" or you wouldn't be eating all the junk you eat. You wouldn't put bad gas in your car on purpose would you? So why do you keep putting bad fuel in your body? That doesn't mean you can't enjoy some of your favorite junk foods or even your favorite fast-food now and then, notice I said **NOW & THEN**, it just means there are no bad foods on the planet ... just a **whole lot of them** you shouldn't eat very often!

Food is universally comfortable. Across the planet, every time any number of people gets together, eating always comes up. From every house, community, tribe, village, town or city – you name it; we go to food as a primary social event. That's what early man did. We grunted and groaned over the first wholly mammoth of the season, we hung out around the fire and told stories about the hunt. Early man was judged by early women on how good of a hunter he was if he brought in a nice kill / food (not too dissimilar from today except instead of a mammoth, it's a nice home or new car or private school for the kids). Later on man still used food as a gathering tool to "break bread" together and share a plate to show friendship. What are we taught in school as kids about Thanksgiving ... the pilgrims were starving and having a hard time in those first years before the Indians helped out and taught them how to hunt the area and catch the fish ... later a gathering happened and that was the first Thanksgiving. Even now, we still use food as a major way of celebrating events and holidays and making peace. As a kid, didn't you get a cookie or some snack, like ice cream, as a reward for doing some chore or getting something done or to pick you up if you were in a funk? When you're sick, you get chicken soup, when you get your tonsils taken out, you get ice cream, when the weather gets cold in Texas, people make chili, in Louisiana they make gumbo, east coasters might do chowders. When a new baby shows up, friends and family bring tons of food. When someone dies, the neighborhood and friends bring enough food for a small army. When early explorers would run into a new group of people in the jungle, if THEY weren't the dinner, then other food was brought out and they were expected to eat with the people of the tribe. Two people cross paths in the desert; they will break bread together, guaranteed!

Why is it that the kitchen ends up being the most popular place to hang when you go to a party? Think about it ... more family problems were hashed out and solved, vacations were planned, businesses started, colleges picked out, weddings were worked on, games were played ... at the kitchen / dining table. And food was served *every single time!* We do a **LOT** of socializing around food!

Food is also the greatest obstacle to most people when starting a fitness routine. Contrary to popular belief, when you do start a new fitness plan or just getting started in fitness period, **DO NOT** start with changing your eating first. Yes, you read that correctly, don't change your eating habits first ... start with the new program, move your body and get used to it and how IT feels first. Reason being, when you start a new physical routine, you're pushing the body harder than before and burning more calories than before, then at the same time you're restricting calorie intake ... something's gotta give! Your body is already going to be stressed from the new exercise and then you're trying to cut back on your fuel intake at the same time you need that extra fuel to do the new work?? That's crazy talk!! Move your body FIRST and get used to that before you start cutting back on the calories. You'll find out real quick that as your body gets familiar with exercise, some of the foods you used to crave wont effect you the same way and you'll be able to reduce or eliminate them from your diet all together. If you're already an experienced exerciser ... same advice, start by getting the body used to the feel of your advanced or new routine *then* work on the new eating that you plan on doing. I promise you, the eating will be a lot easier to do when your body is used to the new work. Just like I said a bit back; if you start cutting back on your nutrition first while at the same time trying to do new physical work on fewer calories ... you'll bonk in a heartbeat and then you'll be worse than before you started. Changing your eating habits will be hard enough when the time is right much less starting out in a nutritional deficit. Eating habits are so deeply ingrained; it will take a lot of discipline to make lasting changes, but once your body feels the exercises and starts to get strong, you'll want to eat the right food and it'll taste right and feel right to make the change. You will get to the point where the junk foods you liked before still taste good to you, but you'll be able to control the cravings and not have them as often ... if you don't stop eating them all together. Quick thought; if you think losing weight or losing inches with *just* changing your eating alone is the right way to go ... you're wrong. You gotta move the body, as in exercise, along with good eating to maximize your health.

If you start by cutting nutrition too quickly, you're setting yourself up for failure both in the physical workout AND your eating plan. Don't rush it! It took a while to get to where you are and it may take a while to get to where you want to be, but IT WILL HAPPEN! Start by making small changes and don't stop. You'll see results soon enough. What's that old saying; "How do you eat an elephant, one bite at a time!"

This chapter is about breaking down the myths, from just a simple misunderstanding to the downright stupid claims that modern diet plans want you to believe. So, here's an example of how crazy it's gotten out there about fitness and diets and weight loss plans. Think for a moment; which of the following people gets the most attention in the media or commercials or on the internet or in some gossip magazine ... the markedly fat individual that loses a bunch of weight over a short period, like a summer ... OR the other individual that has maintained a steady and healthy weight by exercising and eating right for several years and / or most of their life? Well the fat individual of course because its somewhat "sensational", but which one is actually the better story to follow ...

the person that has <u>maintained</u> a healthy lifestyle for many years of course, but that won't sell the "fitness junk" you see on TV. Eating a healthy diet and exercising regularly is what everybody says they want, but the vast majority of them want it YESTERDAY so they take shortcuts ... fat burning pills, "energy drinks", extreme fat burning diets, crazy-assed exercises and exercise plans that work in the short term, but are rarely if ever a long term solution. People just don't want to believe that proper health comes with a bit of sweat and eating discipline. Guys and gals, y'all need to commit the following statement to memory and repeat it often; ***the VAST majority of "diet plans" do NOT work for the VAST majority of people, and the plans that do work are almost NEVER a long term solution.***

Don't buy into "quick" and "overnight" diet plans that want you to lose a lot of weight quickly. There's a "gimmick" in there somewhere ... guaranteed! When you hear about a "new and improved" diet plan that promises quick solutions and have cartoon pictures of people losing body fat – that's your cue to run in the opposite direction and look for a better, more realistic solution. The absolute truth is, eating right is the hardest part of weight management, period. More than enough trials and studies *(1)(2)* have shown that eating right and nutritionally correct is as much as 75-80% of your fitness plan. That's how important good fuel is to the body and to your exercise routine! It has been my experience that I can get the biggest, fattest, and dare I say ... laziest person, up and moving, as in going to the gym and exercising, 100x faster than I can put a dent in their eating habits alone.

Gym people and nutritionists talk about "diet plans" or use the word "diet" a lot without telling you what it really means. Now is a great time to review the definition of "diet" – it means simply; the usual food and drink consumed by an organism – person or animal ... that's it! We've changed the definition a bit in the health and fitness world to almost a negative; such as; "you need to go on a diet" or "that diet is not working" or "try MY diet plan" or "this diet plan is too hard to maintain" or "I saw this diet plan in that fitness magazine" or "you know how many movie stars are doing this diet" ... blah blah blah - puke!! Try this, write down ALL the most common names of diet "plans" you've ever heard of (I'd list a few of them here, but then I'd have to pay them something for mentioning their name), there's a bunch of them, right?? Notice how many you can recall, yet the one diet "plan" that you SHOULD know is the simplest and easiest of all – *eat clean as possible and be active!* While it is acceptable that all these plans you wrote down use the basic premise of restricting your total food intake or the intake of one particular food or intake of a particular "set" of foods, and while that makes sense in concept, it HAS to be realistic or it won't last past the "6-8-12 week" period of the plan. SOME of them go a bit too far by making you think that one or another particular food is almost "poisonous" and even farther by making you buy THEIR food along with some crazy exercise routine that is unsustainable long term.

Please don't get so hung up on the "word" diet – KNOW what it means and follow good common sense and you'll find that making smart choices is a lot easier than you think. To follow a "diet" is to follow how you normally eat – so start eating better and you'll be following a better diet. See what I'm saying ... know what the word means and use it correctly in your head and in your speech and you'll start eating better right off the bat. And, talking about making simple, smart choices, if you even sort-of know the nutritional differences between REAL (lean meats, veggies, fruits, grains ...) food and processed (... just add water) foods, then eat more real food than processed food and you're already on your way to better health.

Let me emphasize TWO distinct thoughts;

FIRST – you CANNOT work off a poor diet – period! There isn't enough time in the day for you to do your job, run the kids around, socialize with your pals and get all the other necessary things done that you have to ... AND burn off the calories of all-day-long poor eating! There was an exercise professor at a college that wanted to test what it would take to burn off a normal, average American "diet", nothing crazy like the guy that ate McDonalds every meal for a month ... but just an average intake of *some* healthy and *some* processed and *some* junk food. Now, he was a professor at a college with all the tools at his disposal and he obviously had the knowledge and time to do the experiment. He tracked the calories he took in each day, and then went to the campus gym to burn off those calories. He took his papers with him, graded them, read them, and made his class assignments ... basically worked while he was on the bike or treadmill and whatever other machine he could get on. Sometimes he was there just a couple of hours after his last class and other times he was there much longer. The take home message ... this was an experiment done at a college with all the resources and tools readily available and it was still a big challenge for this professor to get it done. What chance do you have to burn off a poor diet ... the short answer is none.*(1)* You have to make daily small changes in your activity level AND eating. Do more as often as you can, and the changes will happen, but you have to be realistic ... know that it WILL happen, but it might take longer than you think, so start NOW to make those changes and when that vacation or wedding or reunion event comes up, you will be more ready for it than if you sit on your butt and then start moving only a few weeks before to get into that particular dress or suit or bikini. Be smarter than that! I'm not sure where I heard this, but I love it ... "a year from now you'll wish you started today". So ... start NOW, TODAY!

SECOND - you will not be chained to tuna and green salads for the rest of your life once you start a workout program. In fact just the opposite, you'll better appreciate good food and you'll know when it's okay to indulge in your favorite "not so healthy" snack or night out. Of course your eating will change a little at first, it HAS to. Then, depending on your goals and what you want to achieve, as well as the demands you'll be putting on your body when you start to train at a higher than average level, your eating habits could change dramatically. Go slow and enjoy the process. Make a commitment to eat healthy and lean four days out of seven in the beginning, then as you get better at exercising and learn more about good nutrition take it up a notch and go for six days out of seven. Make that last day a "cheat day". Don't go crazy and over do it, but relax a bit and enjoy some of your favorites – that way it's not that you're completely cutting them out; you're just putting them in their rightful place ... and you're EARNING them. Make it a game, hold off from the sweets or other junk food or alcohol as long as you can, then make that last day a reward. It'll feel more like a real treat than just something you grab to stop some craving. It's better to lose fat slow and steady than to lose it fast ... like the commercials want you to believe.

Here's a little known fast food fact from the Olympic world; fast food, and particularly McDonalds, was crazy over-the-top-mondo popular with ALL the athletes at the Rio games in 2016 *(3)(4)(5)*. Now, this is **not** giving YOU or me permission to eat junk food ... I'm just making the point that even world class athletes make room for a "little" junk or "treat" now and then, besides, these athletes have trained their bodies to a point that they metabolize fat WAY more efficiently and way quicker than the rest of us. So, unless you're one of those guys or gals ... keep processed and junk food to an absolute minimum if you want better results from your workouts.

Our bodies are so incredibly forgiving. We abuse them with drugs (not necessarily the illegal ones either), alcohol, lack of sleep, lack of exercise, bad diets, fake "super energy pills and drinks" ... and it just keeps working. You take your car in for an inspection & tune-up every year, why don't you take your body in for a checkup every year & use exercise to stay tuned-up year 'round? You can get extra parts for your car, but that's not so easy to do with your body parts. We would all be better off if instead of trying to keep up with those neighbors that have the new car or TV or swimming pool or ski boat, we kept up with those healthy neighbors that go for a walk or a jog or bike ride or play tennis ... you name it. We all know THAT active couple that's always on the go. They're active and moving and involved some way all the time and not just sitting around the house watching TV, watching other people be active. Let's say this couple does inspire you to get moving and start a program of your own, fantastic, but then when results don't come fast enough, you stop. How far do you think any of us would get if we did the same thing with our jobs or schooling or a relationship – oh wait, a bunch of us do exactly that!! Anyway … you see what I'm saying? You gotta keep at it, and keep going! Okay, back to nutrition basics...

For thousands and thousands of years, our bodies ran on natural and real foods like fish, fawn and fowl … fruits, vegetables, nuts and grains, natural sugars and fats … AND they ran great!! Really it's only been just a bit over 100 years that we have really jacked up our bodies with chemicals and preservatives and synthetic food additives. Add to that the ridiculous lack of physical activity that the majority of us are doing, or NOT doing, and now we as a country, are approaching 36%, that's just over one third *(6)* of our population, that are close to or full-on obese. Our bodies have no idea how to process all of these junk foods and junk additives. In these past 100+ years of modern man messing with the foods we eat, we have more metabolic disease, more sickness, more allergies, more obesity, and more cancers than ever before … because we're smart and health minded??!! Real food is real food and should be eaten like real food. Processed food should be eaten sparingly and on rare occasions, if at all!! Limit your intake of processed foods and see and feel what happens to you, I think you'll be surprised sooner than you think. If an ingredient on a package has 13 letters a dash and a number … it AIN'T a real food, it's some chemical food additive space-age polymer … who the heck knows??

Try this; eat ALL the single ingredient foods you want, on MOST days of the week and really earn that cheat day. What is a "single ingredient" food you might ask? I'm not talking about vitamins and minerals and all of that, what I'm talking about is foods that you can EASILY say what the main ingredient is. Example; what's in fish – FISH. What's in an apple – APPLE? What's in spinach - SPINACH?

What's in a tomato – TOMATO? What's in a chicken breast – CHICKEN BREAST? What's in an orange – ORANGE! See what I'm saying? If you need spell-check, a dictionary, a scientific periodic element chart or a medical reference book to help read a food label, it isn't a natural food! If you go to the store and get a box or a bag and all you have to do is "just add water" and FOOD happens ... that's not *real* food. Having said that, I'll add here that, "dehydrated" foods are real foods that have just had the water / moisture taken out and are good to go as far as I'm concerned. I love camping and backpacking and actually dehydrate my own meals when I'm planning a trip. All you do is add water to those. That is far different than opening a box of "cheesy-whiz-bang-sugar-snackums" and thinking you're eating real food, 'cuz you're not!

You need to learn how to prepare and eat real food for yourself. Try and not fall for some stupid diet plan that has you buying "their" food to lose weight. You know the ones; you order numbers of breakfasts, lunches, dinners and snacks ... they tell us on their commercials that all you have to do is eat their food and you'll lose weight. That's not a REAL plan. What it is is, a VERY short term solution, but you can and should do better than that. Think of it this way; you're not learning anything when you just buy it and eat it like that. Now, what happens when that company goes out of business, or something happens where you don't receive your shipment of meals? Now where are you going to get your food? Where in the process have you learned how to pick out the right food at the grocery store? When, in the process of just ordering your food and having it mailed to you, did you learn how to fix a healthy plate of food? At what point of your buying and eating, did you learn what a healthy plate, proportionally, looks like? Guys and gals, there are a lot of companies out there doing this to y'all, use your head and don't fall for it. Do your homework and learn about the food you're ordering or better yet, learn how to pick out and prepare healthy food for yourself. Now, I realize that working adults with families may have little time to fix dinner and sit down with the family every night. Okay, then do some food prep over the weekends that you can spread out over the next week. Get the "steamable" vegetables in the frozen food area, use the quick brown rice packs, prep a family package of chicken breasts and have real food ready to eat at a moment's notice. In Naked 2 I'll share a lot more ideas, but start easy and go from there. It's all about developing new habits, and better habits make you better and will absolutely change your life.

Okay, now let's talk about the basic components of your food; carbohydrates, proteins and fats. These are "macronutrients" simply meaning BIG nutrients, as opposed to micro-nutrients (small). Every food you eat is made up of carbohydrates, proteins and fats. Your body needs ALL three to operate properly, but not in equal amounts. To make sure you're getting the CLEANEST possible fuel intake, eat a LOT of the single ingredient foods like we talked about earlier.

Your car needs gas, oil and water just like your body needs **carbs, fat and protein**. You honestly can eat anything you want ... as long as you burn the calories you took in, remember the story of the professor, you just want to make sure that you're eating as clean as possible and as often as possible. The cleaner the food you eat, the better it's utilized by the body and the less you have to worry about burning it off. Ok then, let's move on to what the basics of carbs, fats & proteins are. Let's take a look at each of them in a little more detail.

CARBOHYDRATES; "carbs" -

Despite the bad name carbs were getting a bit ago and still get from time to time, they are still incredibly valuable in your eating plan. Some diet plans will still talk bad about carbs instead of educating you on their REAL value and so they have you eliminating them to dumb levels. Do carbohydrates cause you to get fat ... NO!! OVEREATING causes you to get fat. Carbohydrates are still our prime source of energy for the body and brain. Carbohydrates are the body's gasoline. What would you think of your mechanic if he had you limit the amount of gasoline you put in your car every time you went to the pump? How far would you get before you'd have to tank up again? I know that's a bit extreme, but that's what some of these diet plans are saying when they have you greatly limit or remove carbs from your eating.

Our first and main source of energy comes from carbohydrates, which turn into blood sugars or "glucose" when ingested and is stored in the muscles and liver for your next workout. It is the first fuel that the body goes to when it needs energy, it's the PRIMARY fuel of the brain – the brain doesn't use protein or fats, it uses carbohydrates exclusively for its energy source. That's why when you miss a couple of meals or are fasting from eating for whatever reason or when you cut out carbs from your diet, you get that low-glycogen headache. That's also how bodybuilders got the label of being "dunderheaded" when they're close to a competition, they put extreme limits on their carb intake so they get that "ripped" look ... they're lacking carbs and brain energy. Even Arnold Schwarzenegger used to joke about it when he was competing.

Okay then, what are carbohydrates. Carbohydrates come in two basic forms – remember we're keeping this simple; the two basic forms are Complex carbs and Simple carbs.

- COMPLEX carbs are grains, vegetables, oatmeal, whole grain breads (yes, breads, we'll talk about doing them right a little later on), seeds, legumes, brown rice and beans. These ***burn much more slowly and evenly***, giving you steady energy throughout the day. Complex carbs should make up the bulk of your carb intake.
- SIMPLE carbs are basic carbs. These include, honey, jellies, syrup, candies and soft drinks. These ***burn quickly*** and give you the high and the crash, with ZERO nutrition benefit – empty calories. Simple carbs should be limited with all due haste. Its so freaking hard to get away from sugar these days, but it is do-able and should be a priority on your list of foods

to cut down on for your new eating plan. Just cutting back on sugars will be a huge bonus for you. You'll see AND feel the results quickly. Natural sugars in real food is one thing, just do the best you can at cutting back or eliminating processed foods with added sugars and or adding more sugar to your food yourself. Please see a nutritional professional before making any big changes in your eating, especially if you have any medical issues that may be affected by a sudden change in your day-to-day diet or food intake.

A recommended amount of carbohydrate (4 calories per gram) in your diet really depends on your activity level and goals, but it is generally accepted as 45-65% of your intake. As long as you're active and training, this is a great guideline, but whatever you don't use or burn, any extra carbohydrate / glycogen / sugars is stored in liver, muscle, and fat tissues. In the fitness world, when we say storage we generally mean as fat. So talk with a nutritionist and know what your carb requirements are and stay close to that.

FATS; "lipids"

In medical or chemistry terms, lipids are organic compounds composed mostly of carbon and hydrogen and are essential for cellular health – pretty dry explanation uh? "Lipids" are more commonly called "fats" by the general public. Having said that, know this; while all fats are lipids, not all lipids are fats. I know, confusing, right? Read on.

Fats are important for a number of reasons and ANY diet plan that has you eliminating fat is a bad plan. Fat has an important purpose or better yet, purposes. Fat in your body and in your diet is important for the following reasons – and these are just a few of the many; fat is a secondary source of energy after carbohydrates, fat aids in cellular health, fat is needed for absorption of your fat soluble vitamins: DEAK, fat aids in thermal regulation, fat gives flavor to food – when you smell that steak cooking on the grill, that's not the meat you smell, that's the fat, YUM, and fat also gives insulation and cushioning to your organs. Like I said, these are just a few of the many reasons fat is important ... just make sure you're taking in the right kind of fat. Fats also, have the most calories per gram – 9 calories to be exact. Fats are important! You need 20-35% in your diet. The fats you **DO** want in your diet are mono and polyunsaturated.

- MONO-unsaturated fat comes from olive, peanut, sesame seed, canola oils and avocados and are good for lowering your LDL cholesterol without harming your HDL levels.
- POLY-unsaturated fat comes from corn, cotton seed, safflower, sunflower, soybean and fish oil. The fish oil you want is the omega-3 fatty acids. This kind of fat helps in lowering both LDL *AND* HDL levels ... so watch your intake and limit this fat. Mackerel, salmon, albacore tuna, and sardines are full of omega-3's.

The fats you **DON'T** want in your diet, or at least limit them with all due haste, are; (7)(8)

- Saturated fats; mainly animal fat – meats such as beef, lamb and veal, poultry, whole milk and cheese are full of it. Also some oils like; coconut, palm and vegetable shortenings. Saturated fats are useful in the production of making some body hormones, but as a whole should be avoided as much as possible.
- Trans fats; are made when good fats like polyunsaturated fats are changed by hydrogenation. That's a process where hydrogen is added to liquid oils and turns them into a solid, like grandma's lard and margarine. They came into being to increase the shelf life of baked goods and other foods. Trans fat was put on the bad list in the early '90's, because

of a Harvard study that found those who were eating high amounts of foods with trans fats were twice as likely to have a heart attack than those that ate little to no trans fat. The other thing that trans fats do is lower the good cholesterol and raise the bad – yikes!!!! Read your food labels and when you see "partially hydrogenated oil" ... that's trans fats!!

When looking at foods with or you're thinking of adding and cooking with oils and fats, try to reduce as much as you can the amount of saturated and trans fat as possible. Take home message here ... learn to read food labels!

PROTEINS; "the real body builders"

Proteins are in the body in all kind of ways. Your hair, bones, tendons and ligaments, muscles, cartilage, nails, teeth, and skin are all full of proteins. Protein consists of amino acids. These amino acids are the building blocks that make up protein. Proteins primary function (as far as fitness is concerned) is to build and repair tissue that has been broken down due to exercise. That's why proteins are known as the rebuilder and repairer of the body. Out of the 20 or so amino acids, nine of these are classified as "essential", meaning the body has to have them, but cannot make them itself. You have to get these essential amino acids from the outside – the food you eat. You should be getting 12-15% of your diet in the form of quality proteins. Some examples of sources of quality protein are; meat, fish, dairy, legumes, nuts and seeds. Yes, if you really want to, you can "drink" your protein in the form of shakes and all, but keep in mind that smoothies and protein shakes can be very calorically dense. Fluids set the cessation button in the belly way higher than real food ... meaning if you're drinking a lot of shakes to get your protein in, or you're drinking them as a meal replacement or whatever else you have in mind, you may actually be consuming more calories than with a healthy well-rounded plate of real food. Different proteins to be familiar with are;

Complete proteins – (animal products) contain sufficient amounts of <u>all</u> essential amino acids.

Incomplete proteins – (non-animal or "plant" products) do not. Incomplete proteins lack one or more of the essential amino acids. YOU have to have BOTH for proper health and tissue repair.

Where will you get these complete and incomplete proteins? Animal products contain complete proteins. The down side ... animal products also contain high levels of saturated fats. Look for lean animal products such as; chicken (of course), turkey, egg whites, seafood (be sure you're not allergic) and some of your low fat / no fat (fat free) dairy products. Soy, believe it or not, is the ONLY plant food that is a complete protein by itself. The rest of the plant world contains incomplete proteins, but can be combined to create complete proteins. i.e. beans and rice, peanut butter and bread. Plant products are generally considered healthy and should be included in a balanced diet. Examples of foods high in incomplete protein include nuts, beans, legumes, rice and grains. Though these foods don't contain all the essential amino acids when eaten by themselves, they can still be used by the body to obtain all of the essential amino acids when combined with different foods that are also sources of incomplete proteins.

Guys and gals, don't make eating or planning meals a "chore", just know the difference between real food and processed foods, then, eat more real food than processed food and you're halfway there. We've already discussed that you can eat anything you want ... as long as you burn the calories you eat. Look at this simple chart, put together by a nutritionist friend of mine Sarah E. Yes, it's really simple – it's supposed to be, but it makes a clear point.

Calories IN < Calories OUT → Lose Weight
Calories IN > Calories OUT → Gain Weight
Calories IN = Calories OUT → Maintain Weight

Simple as it is, this makes a fairly clear visual for seeing what food / calories, can do to you or for you if eaten in moderate and appropriate amounts!

The take home message here is to eat "real" food as often as possible and keep the processed food to a minimum. Putting clean fuel in your tank will pay off in your energy levels, your brain power, your rest and recovery! If you're an organism that needs to eat, then eat clean.

(1) http://www.mayoclinic.org/healthy-lifestyle/nutrition-and-healthy-eating/basics/nutrition-basics/hlv-20049477

(2) http://www.womenshealthmag.com/weight-loss/weight-loss-80-percent-diet-20-percent-exercise

(3) https://www.washingtonpost.com/world/the_americas/olympic-athletes-are-gorging-themselves-on-free-mcdonalds/2016/08/12/25f0eb35-5a26-4bdb-8643-123855fb0430_story.html?utm_term=.3574b6ad622d

(4) http://time.com/4453092/mcdonalds-rio-olympic-village-2016-olympics/

(5) http://www.newsweek.com/rio-olympics-athletes-eating-mcdonalds-490813

(6) https://www.cdc.gov/obesity/data/adult.html

(7) http://www.webmd.com/cholesterol-management/guide/understanding-numbers#1

(8) http://www.webmd.com/diet/guide/understanding-trans-fats

The WRAP:

- Food IS fuel
- Do not change your eating habits AND start a new strenuous routine.
- The vast majority of diets do not work for the vast majority of people, and the ones that do work are almost never a long term solution.
- Your BEST diet plan is to eat clean AND be active.
- You cannot work off a poor diet.
- Eat more "real" food.
- Eat as little "processed" food as possible.

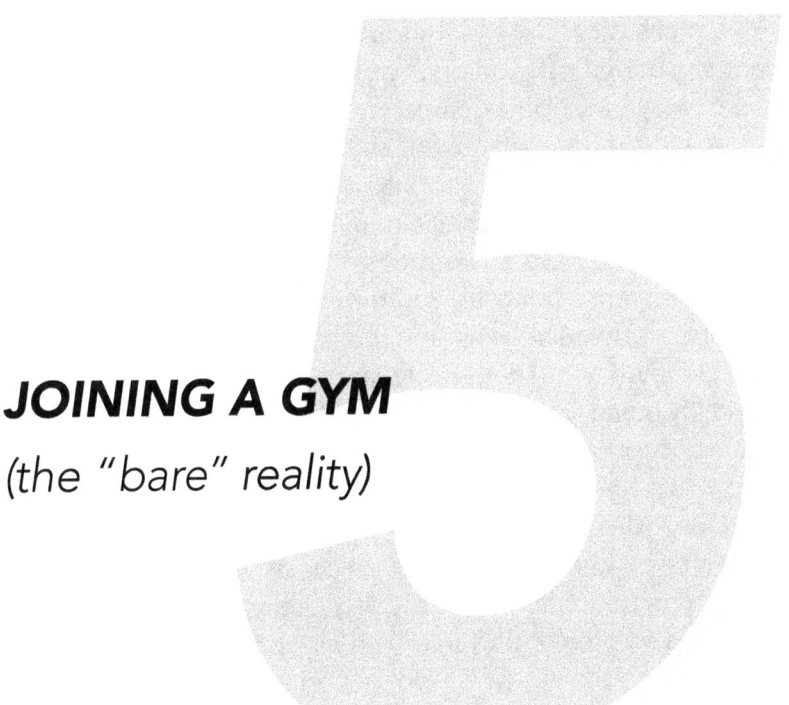

JOINING A GYM

(the "bare" reality)

Okay, now that you know more how to define "fitness" and know a few of its important benefits and are practicing some solid nutritional basics ... let's talk about joining a gym, if that's what you want to do. First off, don't just go to the local gym because that's where everybody else is going. Find a gym that suits you personally. Nowadays almost every town, even a small one, has a choice in gyms, from the mom and pop family gym to a chain gym; you will more then likely have a choice to make. That's to your advantage!! You're going to have to like going to that gym. That alone could be the difference between you getting up and getting in a good workout on a regular basis, and the days you'd rather skip just 'cuz it's a cloudy day or some other lame excuse. If you like the place and enjoy going, you won't skip out. Make sure the atmosphere, the lighting, the music, the staff ... make sure you're good with all of it. I know sometimes you won't "see" all of the gym until you've been there for a while, so ask for a trial period. A lot of gyms will give you as much as a week to try out the place as well as the classes. The thing to do now is to ... actually **TRY** the gym out! Go to as many classes as you're comfortable with visiting, use the showers, use the "kids club" if you have a kid, get on every piece of equipment, talk to other members ... but, if you walk in and honestly don't like something or if it doesn't feel right, walk out. You're not obligated, so get out of there and go check out another gym. Another way to do this is to go as a guest with a friend to their gym. This way you also get his/her inside knowledge of the place, and they'll show you around so you do not have to figure it out on your own.

In Naked Fitness 2 we'll go into much more detail about setting and reaching personal fitness goals, but for now, start with small achievable goals and work your way up to the bigger ones, make your gym goals small and very achievable as well. Start small and build from there. Get used to your new routine. Try different times and different days to see what works best for your energy level and schedule. If you joined with a friend then "practice" a few days and times to see what works best for the two of you. Working out with a friend also does wonders for your encouragement and accountability.

When you do join a gym the important thing here (yes, I'll say it one more time) is ... to **GO!** There have been studies *(1)* that have shown the average gym member would actually save money on their monthly gym dues if they just paid the visitor fees every time they showed up. That's pretty sad, you join a gym and then waste the money not showing up. The point is to **SHOW UP!** Start slow and start easy. Get used to the place and the routine of the gym. **You** joined it, it didn't join you. And please don't start out like some crazy-gonna-change-my-life-overnight-fanatic person going every day and staying for hours at a time. You'll overdo it and get hurt and then you'll really not go back. I know it's awkward and you don't want to be seen as a new person not knowing where everything is, but I'm here to tell you, people will notice more that you're a newbie to that particular gym and a newbie to exercise too, if you act like you're not. You'll learn more, have more fun and meet more people if you ask questions and you'll get more help and you'll enjoy the place more if you don't act like you've been there forever. Believe me, regular members will know that you're new no matter what you do, so just get in there and ask questions.

If you're not a regular exerciser and not completely comfortable in a gym then just go once, walk around and try out the locker room and a few machines and then leave. Wait a day or two then go again and try a different piece of equipment. Then ask what classes they offer or look at a schedule that most gyms post just for that reason. Look for a class that you might know of or one that sounds familiar or the one your friend was talking about etc. If you don't like it, don't go back, try a different class. Then later you can circle back and try that same class and you just might find out that you do actually like it. Members that have been at a gym for years, stop going to a class and try a different one from time to time, it's ok. You get the idea, you gotta' start somewhere. Even in a class that you are familiar with but haven't been in a long time, start slow and progress as you feel stronger / better and at a pace that won't hurt you. It's a much safer plan for your body and mind that you start easy and make smooth and steady progress. Your body will thank you and your mind wont stress trying to get too far ahead of the goals you set. Now, let's say you do get into it right off the bat. You like the gym and the members you've met. The classes are fun and you want more, ok then, go for it! Keep in mind all the previous information still holds even for you at this stage. Slow and steady wins the day. It just means that you'll be in better shape sooner because you're really enjoying the process and you'll stick with your goals.

Other basic exercise guidelines you'll want to consider; always warm-up before a workout. All you need is five to ten minutes of a medium walk or jog. Stretch your major muscle groups, chest, back and legs. You need to warm-up even if you're going to do a cardio workout. Warming up the body does exactly that, it heats up the body and loosens muscles and joints so you can work them with less chance of injury. Everyone needs to do a proper warm-up. Don't be one of the guys or gals that don't do a proper warm-up. You know the ones out there that are always hurting or getting injured from their activities. I'll bet a lot of them, one; don't warm-up correctly or enough, and two; deep down they probably think a "proper" warm-up and stretching is for someone else, not them – how stupid! Olympians warm-up and stretch, they ALWAYS do a "prep" routine before their workouts ... and you should too. Don't let your buddy, who's always hurt and aching and **NOT** doing a proper warm-up, and seeing a doctor for his / her pains, tell you that a warm-up is a waste of time. I hope we're all smarter than that, but there are still a LOT of those guys and gals out there ... don't be one of them!! We'll go a LOT deeper into this in Naked Fitness 2.

The take home here is, if you join a gym ... USE IT!!!

(1) http://www.ptdirect.com/training-design/
exercise-behaviour-
and-adherence/attendance-adherence-drop-ou
t-and-retention-patterns-of-gym-members

The WRAP:

- Look at every gym you can and pick the one that fits YOU.
- Take advantage of a "trial" period.
- Then GO to the gym.
- Try different times and days to better set your routine.
- Start slow but steady.
- Look for Naked Fitness 2 to learn more about working out.

FINDING A TRAINER

(the "naked" essentials to finding a "well dressed" trainer)

Now, if you decide that you need help and you really want to try a personal trainer ... let's find you one. Here are a few tips and additional information related to finding a top notch trainer. There are several benefits to hiring a personal trainer to help you with your fitness goals. The first of which is, in my opinion, the most important – **adherence**. You won't get ANY benefit if you don't stick to any program, especially the program that you're paying for. With your hard earned money on the line you're more likely to show up and do the work. You could get a 10x gold medal Olympic winning coach to make up a workout program for you that's guaranteed to work, but if you don't do it, how much help is it?

A few other benefits are;

1. **Accountability** – you're answering to someone for your exercise time.
2. **Motivation** – from your trainer and from your own results. When you see it working, you'll work harder.
3. **Personalized programs** – if your trainer is doing his/her job, your workout is LITERALLY made for you and only you. Everyone has arms and legs and does the same basic exercises, but how specific exercises are put together in the right sets and reps as it relates to you and your body and needs and physical goals is how it becomes truly personal.
4. **Supervision** – checking form and body posture is very important when weight or strength training. Again, if your trainer is doing their job then every movement you make is being watched and analyzed. What good is it to do an exercise that's not being supervised to make sure you're getting the best out of it or if you're doing it wrong and they're not watching to see if it could hurt you – that's not what you're paying for; you **are** paying for his/her supervision. Don't be afraid to remind them of this if you have too.

Now, here are a few thoughts about how to go about picking your trainer. The real world truth is you won't know how good or how bad they really are until you get involved, so consider these tips before you make a decision on one.

First thing to do is to watch all the trainers in your gym. Watch how they each interact with their clients. Watch to see if they're paying attention to how their clients do the exercise and if they're coaching them along, being engaged in the exercise with the client or are they "leaning" on another machine or sitting on the floor telling the client what to do. Watch to see if they are texting or looking at the television or eating/drinking something and talking to other trainers or members. You DON'T want that trainer … period! A **LITTLE** of that is totally acceptable, you DO want a trainer that has a bit of personality, but it'll be obvious when it's too much and too often. I just said it above, a good part of the service you're paying for is your trainer's _attention_. They should be attentive and focused … on you!

Next, you might want to ask around to see if any of your friends or another gym member knows of a good trainer or even uses one and whom. Referrals say a lot – most of the time. Then take the time to watch that particular trainer and how they train their clients. No trainer escapes a buyer's gaze no matter what their clients say about them. The clients are obviously biased to that trainer so they may not view him/her the same way you will as a new potential client. Ask your friend or gym member why they use that particular one. A good starting point for you might be to find a trainer that specializes in something you like; golf, tennis, running or swimming. They don't necessarily have to be a "champion competitor" in that area, but if they are then all the better. Most likely when a trainer specializes like that, they do have experience in that sport or activity. You'll be fine. Any way you slice it, a respectable trainer will still be of great value to your fitness life.

Once you pick a trainer, you'll want to interview him/her. This must be as thorough of an interview as if you're an employer interviewing a potential employee ... cuz that's exactly what's going on; you're hiring them to work for you. See how that works? Don't hold back on the information you want to know about him/her. Be confident in asking what experience they have, what certifications they have, what they think their best training attribute is, what their training philosophy is – and they should be able to answer this one! If they stutter and stammer to find an answer or if they say anything that makes you look at them like a dog that hears a weird noise, don't walk away – RUN and find another trainer to visit with. A reputable trainer will have a solid philosophy to their training. In the end, it doesn't matter what the reason is, you still have the right to walk away if you don't like what you're hearing or feeling with this particular person, remember, you're going to have to be with this person every week for a specific amount of time. You're going to give this person a good chunk of your hard earned money. You're about to trust this person with your health. You're going to have to like them to a certain degree. You have to trust your gut feelings.

Next, you definitely want someone that has at least one NATIONALLY recognized certification. Some of these include; NSCA – National Strength and Conditioning Association. ACSM – American College of Sports Medicine, NASM – National Academy of Sports Medicine, The Cooper Institute – in Dallas, Texas. There are plenty more certifications out there; these are just some of the best in the business. Look on your favorite web-browser, "compare personal training certifications", and you will get a lot of info to go through. Now, just because the trainer you picked might have one of the certifications listed and maybe even a degree in exercise, that doesn't mean you're going to get the results you want or even get the kind of service that you were promised in the interview you had with him/her, but it gives you a baseline of expertise and professionalism that you should expect from a trainer with that certification or degree.

Next, you'll definitely want a trainer that is insured and bonded, so ask; do they have liability insurance? Insurance protects him/her, the gym and you, so it's important to know if they carry any. If they say something like "no, the gym covers me." That's fine and the gym really might be covering their trainers, but a trainer that goes the extra mile and has his/her own liability insurance is a trainer confident in their skills and one that puts personal responsibility high on the list. This is the trainer you want! Are they CPR or some other first-aid certified? Nowadays virtually any certification worth their weight will require CPR training as well. Some won't even give out a certificate if you don't have a valid CPR card – that's a good thing! Next, it certainly isn't required, but ask if they happen to have a small list of clients they might allow you to contact for additional reference. Again, this is a trainer confident in his/her ability. Remember though, trust what you SEE not what you're told, even by their current clients.

Money has to come up sometime so, ask how much they charge and if they offer some "bulk sessions" or special promotions. Some gyms handle all of the money and the trainer has very little if anything to do with making special deals, but it doesn't hurt to ask. If the trainer is an independent contractor they will be able to make a deal with you, but as an independent they also have the right to charge you whatever the market can bear, so ask BEFORE you sign up! Ask if you can you work with a friend and get a package deal or bulk sessions at a good price as well?

Let's talk about "price" for a second. Please don't get caught up in the myth that the more you pay the better the trainer will be. Spending more money than you should, won't guarantee you any quicker or better results. I've met trainers with a national certification and an appropriate degree and couldn't put a two car parade together. And then, I personally know several really smart and careful trainers that have a quality certification and nothing more than experience and they get results! It's like any other profession, some are good, some are great, and some you wouldn't use if they were offering free services. It is my personal opinion that unless you're a paid, competitive athlete, meaning, you are making money from a sport or competition that the trainer is a big part of, NO trainer is worth $100.00 or more per session! If you feel it's important for you to spend that kind of money because your friend is, or your friend set you up with that particular trainer and you don't want to look cheap ... then go for it, lucky trainer, but it still guarantees you nothing. Do your homework and use your head. Think of it this way ... your trainer is going to make you run, do crunches, jump rope, lift weights, push and pull tires and who knows what else, but ... it's not life or death or front line combat, so it shouldn't cost you an arm and a leg, but it should be "valuable", in that you get real value for what you're paying. If you feel, during any session, like the trainer is "phoning it in" ... let them know right then and there and if it happens again, fire them and get someone else. It's up to you.

Now, keep in mind that the "interview" you do with your trainer isn't ALL on him or her, part of it is up to you as well, make sure you give a complete and honest history of any exercise and or injury issues that might interfere with the training he/she might provide. I have an opinion (oh please, not another one) on trainers that blow through or even blow off taking a thorough history of your past aliments and exercise. Every certification I can think of requires the trainer to take a good history. That's the only way your trainer will know how to put together a proper and correct personal exercise plan. If you went to see a new doctor and he/she just started throwing medications at you without getting a good medical history, you'd probably turn him/her in for malpractice. There is no difference here. You **want** your trainer to know about you and your "exercising past". That way they know what exercises to pick to strengthen or stretch or leave alone to re-balance you. Another point; almost any activity will at some point pull or push a body part just a bit too far. When that happens most of us ice and massage it and elevate it for say, oh I don't know ... *2 MINUTES*, and think all is well. You're going to "favor" that part and sooner or later you'll develop an imbalance if you're not really careful. If your trainer doesn't take time to do a thorough history on you, how thorough do you think he/she will work through and develop your exercise prescription? Think about it.

Picking a time for both of you can sometimes be a deal breaker. I've lost potential clients when after sailing easy through everything else; we couldn't find a time we both agreed on. You want to make sure to go in with a pretty solid idea of your first, second and third best times of the day that would work for you as well as the first, second and third best days of the week that would work for you to meet with this person. They might be booked on your first choice so you want to be sure to have more times ready to go to. Trainers should work around YOUR schedule first ... and if for some reason that doesn't work then you'll have to see what else they have available. Y'all work it out together.

Once you've made up your mind on a trainer to meet with, you've met and set a time and day to train and have agreed on money ... then have a blast and get fit! A good trainer who's really watching out for you and keeps you motivated is truly invaluable when it comes to your health and fitness. He/she should be keeping records of your progress and you definitely want them to do that for you, don't fall for the "waiter" kind of trainer. As much as I like a good waiter that remembers my order and all the extras, it doesn't work that way with your health, so you shouldn't accept any trainer telling you something like "...it's okay, I'll remember all your workouts and your progress". Don't bet on it! As old fashion as it sounds, you'd be better served by a trainer that carries a clipboard with your workout on it – that's a record that both you and the trainer should have access to at a moment's notice. You want to see your progress as well, right?

Next thing ... DON'T miss your appointments!!! The whole reason you're putting your hard earned money on the line is to get results ... well, the obvious is ... you won't get results if you don't show up! A buddy of mine says; "you can't win if you don't play" and it totally applies here, you will not get the results you want if you're not there to do and to learn them. Plus ... you will more than likely get charged for any session you miss if you don't let your trainer know ahead of time. One thing that gets under a trainers skin faster than anything, is when you no-show or miss appointments with little notice. If they're doing their job ... they have planned out your session and are ready to work. Every trainer knows that "crap" happens, but that doesn't give you the right or excuse to waste their time! It's up to your trainer to decide if they'll charge you for a missed session. If you do miss often ... you're going to get charged. If you missed because you slept in ... you'll get charged. If you missed because you just didn't feel like coming in ... you'll get charged. If you woke up and you have a flat tire or the kid is sick or YOU'RE sick, then you probably won't get charged. It's still going to be up to the trainer to decide to charge or not charge you. The take home message here; DON'T MISS YOUR APPOINTMENTS unless it's an honest emergency! Now, you need to ask what the trainer will do for YOU if he/she misses an appointment. That's important to know.

You're going to feel so much better and look great in the process. Once you have a feel for working out, your discipline is established, you have a bank of exercises in your head and if you feel you could actually go off on you own without your trainer; it's perfectly acceptable to take a break and try it on your own for awhile. That's what he/she is really for, to get you going so you can go off on your own and then come back for a tune-up now and then. The "Zen" of a trainer's job is to work themselves out of a job. If they're doing their job right, you learn for a while and then try it on your own. If you like the services they provide, then you stay. The true work of a good trainer is to teach you fitness and then tweak your program and show you something new periodically if you decide to try it on your own. I don't mean to go on so much about using and being careful of working with a personal trainer, but this is one of the biggest areas of fitness where you can get really hurt and or get really ripped off. Hiring a trainer will be rewarding enough if you take the right steps, it shouldn't be a risky endeavor.

The WRAP:

- Hire a trainer if you aren't sure of what you're doing.
- A quality trainer is worth having.
- Watch the trainers at your gym.
- Ask around who the staff AND members think is a good trainer.
- Find one that specializes in your sport or interest.
- Do YOUR homework and don't be afraid to ask a lot of questions.
- Don't miss your appointments.
- Learn from your trainer and then at an appropriate time, stop and try it on your own.

GYM ETIQUETTE

*(the "bare" essentials to being
a decent acting member)*

RULES are good!! We have rules all over the place. Some are posted and some are just implied as the right thing to do. Let's look at some of the rules you run into everyday. On the doors of a restaurant you might see something like – "no shirt, no shoes no service", in the bathrooms you'll see – "employees must wash hands". On a gas pump you'll see – "cash customers please pay first". At the bank or the movies or amusement park you'll see cuing lines with a sign that says something like – "line starts here". At a coffee shop the vast majority of people wait in line for their turn without a whole lot of difficulty. Same thing at the grocery store, you get in a line and stand there until your turn to check out. This isn't difficult to understand and for the most part, we all follow these rules of the establishment we're in. WHY then, do far too many people disregard the rules in a gym??? Why is a gym any different than any other public place that appreciates rules?

Gym members are notorious for "bucking" the rules. And it's not just the guys acting like they own the place ... the gals have exhibited some of the same ridiculous and over-the-top stupid behavior. In a gym I was just recently involved with, an honest to goodness fight almost broke out with a bunch of the ladies because a Pilate's class changed a couple of its procedures in class scheduling. I mean really ... it's the gyms prerogative to change the days or the times or take the thing off the schedule ... IT'S JUST A FREAKING CLASS PEOPLE!!! Staff and trainers won't admit it, but we all really hate it when we also encounter the "elder" crowd when they want to push their way around as well. We absolutely respect their opinion and are happy to see them there and being active, but when an elder / senior member is approached with a rule-concern and they reply with something like (and this has happened to ME personally several times in my career) "... you know how long I've been a member here ...", my response is, "yes, I do know, and that makes it worse because you should know better"! You don't get a free pass on breaking the rules just because you've been a member for a long time or are "old". Come on folks, rules are there for a reason and unless you own the place, just follow the rules no matter how you feel about it. The vast majority of gyms have visible signs up letting you know what the rules are. LOOK for the signs, don't pretend you didn't see it – I've seen this as well, someone wearing flip-flops and standing *right in front* of a sign that says "closed toe gym shoes only on the weight floor" telling me they don't see a sign that says they can't wear them!! Ladies and gents ... if you want to impress the staff or someone else in the gym, set the example and do the right thing ... follow the rules! Again, unless you *own the gym* ... just obey the rules. What makes people think they're so special that they're above the posted rules? The rules of a gym are there for a host of reasons such as, the protection of the gyms equipment, the other members, physical safety and biological safety. You want to make a great impression on your new gym??? Ask them for a list of the rules when you sign up ... and then follow them! I'll go a little further and say, one of the greatest reasons that you see all the craziness in gyms these days is because of the "fad-fitness" programs out there. They teach a lot of bad technique and they teach to move fast and throw things around ... they're like a virus in the world of good and sustainable fitness.

So let's now look at some of the most common and ... most common sense, rules that you **WILL** see in a gym setting and that you should be familiar with.

At the top of **MY** list for this book is;

- **Don't drop weights or slam the machines.**

Now, let me start by saying ... even the most muscle-bound meathead trainer at almost any gym in the country doesn't like it when a "want to be" body builder drops the weights and throws stuff around like some gorilla. NOBODY likes it. Simply put ... unless you **OWN** the gym you workout in, **DON'T DROP THE WEIGHTS OR SLAM THE MACHINES!** I've seen dumbbells get bent, the heads broken off, collars on weight plates get cracked and broken to the point that they have to thrown away ... all because some knucklehead wants the entire gym to know he / she is there and lifting more than they can handle. When you slam the fixed machines, all you're doing is loosening up the connections and cracking the plates and making excess noise, again just so everyone else knows you're there ... WTF!!! You guys (and unfortunately more and more girls) that drop weights are hated by those who really know how to handle weights. All you're doing is impressing the other guy or girl that drops weights and doesn't know what they're doing either ... freaking knock it off! I guess I could be nice about this and say things like "pretty please don't drop the weights" or "you could possibly damage the weights or machines if you drop or slam them down" ... but you already know this so why should your gym or ANY gym politely ask you not to do something you already know? Just STOP doing it all together! If there is no proper "drop floor or platform" or if the weights are not proper "drop weights" then **DON'T DROP THE WEIGHTS!**

I think the best thing I can say about this is ... **REAL** athletes that use weights correctly as tools of fitness, don't "drop" them. They know the value of good tools and consider weights "good tools". Think about it. Learn to lift and set down your weights properly. You'll stay healthier than most, and maybe you can help someone else do it right as well.

- **Keep your grunting and noise making to a minimum if at all.**

It's understandable that when you exert power and energy, you want to forcefully exhale to help the process, there is a lot of science to that ... but keep it to a minimum and keep it low. You don't need to grunt and holler with every rep, that's just stupid. There is **NO** need to sound like you're in some kind of mating season episode on Animal Planet. **NO ONE** wants to hear you grunt and grown – so shut up!!

- **Wipe down the machines and other equipment.**

If you've sweated all over them or even if you haven't, if YOU sat on it, YOU wipe it off. This should be a no-brainer, but the simple rule is, wipe off the machines *whenever* you use one. It's not just the machines and benches … if you sweated all over a floor mat, wipe it off. If you sweated all over a physio-ball, wipe it off. If you left a pool of sweat under a cycle / spinner bike, it's a good bet you've sweated all over the bike itself, wipe it off! **NO ONE** wants to sit on a bench, or use a mat or a ball or ride that bike, with your sweat all over it. I don't care how precious you think your sweat is … no one else does!!

- **Put back weights and ANY other equipment YOU took off a rack or a stand**

If you used a jump rope, a medicine ball, a physio ball, any cable handles, battle ropes … if you used it or you got it out, you put it back. Yes guys and gals, almost every gym in the country has "floor staff" that picks up equipment and puts things away and cleans the equipment … but that doesn't make them your maid or personal servant. Put on your big boy undies and your big girl panties and clean up after yourself!

- **Wear proper gym shoes**

This means closed toe SNEAKERS, not sandals, loafers, crocks, socks, cowboy boots or muddy workboots, common sense here folks. I know, sometimes you forget and you're stuck with what you have – whatever that is, so, here's a cool little fix for that … keep an old pair of sneakers in your car just in case. Problem solved.

- **Wear appropriate gym clothes**

Again, think about it; don't wear jeans, casual slacks, ratty ass cut t-shirts or shorts or a t-shirt that has been cut from the underarm down to the waistband ... really??? You might think you're "being an individual and you aren't going to be told how to dress" too bad, every gym is different, but if you don't **own** the gym ... just follow the rules.

- **Use a proper water bottle**

Use one that has a sport tip on it or at least a closable lid and not just an open cup of water you're carrying around. Oh, while we're here ... there's this really cool thing in gyms these days called "water fountains" where you can get as many drinks of cool water as you want ... so why do some of you feel it's necessary to carry around a gallon jug of water? Don't be a tool! Use a big sport bottle and go fill it up when it's empty, what's the big deal?

- **How about wash your hands after you use the bathroom.**

Yeah, you know you've done it ... that's just gross. You might think you're the only one not washing your hands, but take a wet hand towel and wipe it across one of the bars on the bench press or even dumbbell handles ... then get ready to be nauseous. Just think of all the other members that think THEY are the only ones not washing their hands after they go potty. How the heck do you think that's appropriate?? While we're talking about the bathroom ... guys, what is y'alls problem ... flush the freaking commode and urinal!! I mean, especially the urinal ... the handle is right in front of you!! Do you not flush the commode at home?? And while we're in the locker-room, clean up around the sink when you get through shaving. Do you leave your sink at home with shaving cream and whiskers all over the counter ... I don't think so. And if you do, that's YOUR house, DON'T do it at the gym.

- **Unload the weight machines when you get done.**

Just be a good member and re-rack you're your weights. Even if there were weights on the machine when you got there, if you lifted them, you put them up. Your momma or your nanny doesn't work for the gym. Do it yourself.

- **Keep your cologne and perfume to a minimum.**

This one is for both you guys and gals, if you're serious about your workouts, put on some deodorant for your body and chew some gum for your breath and leave the cologne and perfume for after you're done with your workout and cleaned up! Few things are more nauseating then when you're sweating and working out and somebody gets next to you that has on enough cologne or perfume to choke a horse!! If you're wearing that much cologne or perfume ... what other "stink" are you hiding or are you thinking of "picking up" something else besides the weights ... really???

There are lots of other rules that may be more "locally important", but if you follow this simple list, you will be a very well liked member at your gym by the staff AND other members ... promise!!

This was a really short chapter ... because it should be common sense. You guys know this stuff, but you let those hayseeds in the gym influence you to do dumb stuff, turn it around and influence them to do it the right way.

The WRAP:

- LEARN the correct way to lift and set down your weights.
- KNOW the rules of your gym.
- PRACTICE the rules of your gym.
- Unless you own the gym ... FOLLOW the rules of the gym.
- PASS on what you learn.

GYM VOCABULARY

(the "bare" truth of what you're saying)

This chapter is devoted to some of the most common terms and slang that you'll hear in a gym. You want to know what they really mean, because a lot of them get used wrong by guys and gals that know what they're talking about, but might be using the wrong word – term – definition. Why is this important? Mainly because I love education and I hate it when I hear people using the wrong terms to explain things. It's a pet peeve of mine!

Okay, here we go. Here are some of the most common "gym" terms you'll hear or maybe you've heard and don't know exactly what they mean. Some of these might seem "old fashioned", I don't care; they're still easy to understand and relative, so here we go.

- **Sets and reps;** "sets" are just groups of repetitions (reps), typically the average exerciser is looking to do two to three sets of 10 to 15 reps each set. Obviously this is goal dependant and will vary with each person, but it's a good place to start if you haven't exercised for a while. Keeping within the scope of this book, keeping it really really simple and not giving you individual strength plans (that'll be in Naked Fitness 2), you'll need to see a trainer for more information. Refer to Chapter 6.
- **Super-set;** this is doing exercises for two or more different body parts (chest and back or back and legs or bicep / triceps ... any combination) back to back in quick succession. I still hear this one being used and still think it makes sense to say that you are doing a "super-set" when doing exercises like this. It's not **that** old school, is it?
- **Compound sets;** this is doing two or more exercises for the same body part back to back in quick succession. Say, a bench press and a dumbbell fly would make a basic compound set. A seated back / lat pull-down with a rowing or back extension exercise would make another combination. Doing a set of squats then lunges and maybe even a hamstring exercise back to back would make a good leg compound

set. You could add any number of exercises to a single body part to make it a really tough compound set.

- **Hypertrophy;** pronounced "hi-purr-trah-fee", is a fancy word meaning growth, so ... muscle hypertrophy is muscle growth, not necessarily "getting huge", just muscle growth in general.
- **Core and / or Core Training;** one of the most **OVERUSED** words / terms in fitness. Seasoned fitness people still throw these around because that's all they've heard it called or afraid to sound too different than normal or to sound like they know what they're talking about to people that don't know what they're talking about, and new people to exercise say it because they aren't really sure what it means, but it sounds cool. I'm certain to ruffle feathers from the fitness group, but hey, they too are in the education business and should be telling their clients and class students the right terms and what they really mean.

I'll make this very simple and not many people will argue with you if use this explanation. Most people will tell you the core is your stomach / abs and maybe some area of your low back. They are correct, but only a little. The *core* of the body is actually the "center" of the body, just like the core of an apple, but the ***trunk*** is from your hips to shoulders – I tell my clients to stop saying and thinking "core" and to start saying and thinking "TRUNK". This is what I teach my clients and anyone who asks. Don't ever say "core" again, its trunk! Exercise science is always tweaking this subject, but without a doubt when you think about where you bend and twist and where your "mass" is, it's from the hips to the shoulders. That's your trunk. **ALL** movement beyond just limb movement, is done with and through the trunk, that's why I push "trunk" work with ALL my clients. When you trunk train you're doing twisting, bending, flexing and extending exercises that make **ALL** movement stronger and more stable. The hips and shoulders are ball joints. In their beauty is their detriment. They are beautiful in that they move in the unlimited range of motion that they do. Their detriment is that they move in the unlimited range of motion that they do. Most other joints are hinge joints or a variation of a hinge. They are somewhat "fixed" in their employment in that they only move as a hinge or move in a limited fashion. Your trunk contains reproductive system, digestive system, circulatory and respiratory systems. Everything else is a limb or a head. The arms feed and push and pull things to and away from the trunk, while the legs move all of the above. The correct way to train your body is from the trunk OUT to the limbs and not from the limbs IN to the trunk. That's why some type of trunk training should be done by everyone in every workout. I'll have a full trunk program in book 2.

- **Weight training versus strength training;** if you're into splitting hairs, you're going to like this subject as well. Ok, this is how I explain the two of these to my clients and people that ask. Yes, you absolutely gain strength when you lift weights but you don't have to lift weights to gain strength. (I'm cracking my knuckles over the keyboard) Here we go; to literally "weight" train, that is exercise training with weights, you gotta use weights, you with me here? Please do not think that I'm making fun of you or anyone else, but I have literally had this very conversation with far more people than I should have! How else can you "bench press" if you're not using a bench and a barbell? How would you do "cable" fly's without a cable machine? How would you do a traditional "leg press" without a leg press apparatus? How would you do a "dumbbell" press without using dumbbells? Now, don't go and get all in a huff over this. All I'm saying is if you're lifting actual **weights** of any kind in any fashion, in an attempt to get stronger or bigger muscles, then you are **weight** training. I am NOT saying these aren't valid and awesome exercises, I am saying you don't need them to gain strength. To strength train you can lift weights, sure, or you can lift your body as in traditional strength exercises – good ol' military physical education, push-ups, pull-ups, plyometrics, agility drills ANY exercise that puts stress on the muscles in an attempt to "grow" them. MOVING THE BODY like in the real world, will make you strong and lean and burn fat, which is the goal anyway right?

- **Cardiovascular training;** all movement, and any exercise for that matter, will touch on your cardiovascular (heart and blood circuit) system. To be more specific, to exercise your cardiovascular system is to do exercises that target that system. Walking, running, swimming, rowing, biking ... are all high quality movements and exercise, but none of them will make your muscles grow like weight or strength training. They certainly will test and tax your muscles and therefore promote growth in more of a muscle endurance way, not so much in the hypertrophy way. For good health and muscle balance you need to do all three; cardio, weight and strength training.

- **Interval Training;** you can split cardio exercise into two basic groups; "steady state" and "interval". Steady state is just that, a pace that's nice and steady and doesn't change much if at all. Think of jogging at a steady and regular pace. You can bike, walk, swim, etc., at a steady and regular pace for endurance and steady calorie burning. Intervals are exercising at a slower pace for a bit of time then amping it up and moving faster for a bit of time and then returning back to your slower pace. Think of walking for two-three minutes, then jogging quickly for one-two minutes, then returning to your slower pace for two-three minutes and repeating as many times as you want. This kind of training works with all the exercises mentioned above; walking, swimming, biking, rowing, etc. You can change the times of intervals to reflect your fitness level or the goals you are trying to reach. At the end of this chapter, I've included a sample interval workout plan that you can fit to just about ANY cardio exercise. If you need help with understanding it better, ask a trainer at your gym. They should be able to help.

- **Tabata:** A type of high intensity interval training. This training protocol involves performing a particular exercise (or exercises) at high intensity for 20 seconds followed by 10 seconds of rest. This is repeated eight times for a total training time of four minutes. You could perform the same exercise for each of the eight 20-second intervals or you could perform a series of different exercises to create a four-minute circuit training type of workout. You could also repeat the four-minute Tabata cycle for multiple sessions. Typically, four sets of "Tabatas" are recommended with one minute of rest time in between each set for a total of a 20-minute workout. More on this type of training and how to use it effectively in Naked Fitness 2.

- **Fitness assessment;** is a very concise and compact set of fitness exercises / tests that will tell your trainer or evaluator about your strengths & weaknesses as well as where and how you're imbalanced. A smart and quality trainer will always do an eval on a new client and then again down the road at some point with their regular clients to see how they have improved. In Naked Fitness 2, I give you my fitness assessment that I use with my clients, along with a couple of other tests. Try it and see what you think. You can contact me if you have any questions.

There are a LOT more to learn, this is just a few of the basics to get you started. Do your own homework and study what you're doing. Don't let someone just tell you how to workout. You may need a push, we all do, but after that, do your own homework. Remember; someone can give you a fish and you'll eat for a day, but if you learn to fish, you'll eat for a lifetime!

Okay, now onto the Interval Program I've included. This particular outline is easily adjustable to ANY paced cardio exercise you can think of. Follow the numbers and see what you think. All you'll need to know your Resting Heart Rate and have a calculator. Then add your numbers in the formula and give it a shot.

Heart Rate Zone Formula:

220 – age = A
A – resting heart rate = B
B x .50 + add back resting heart rate
.60"
.70"
.80"
.90"

Let's see this worked out with a person that's 40 years old and a resting heart rate of 55.

220 – 40 = 180
180 – 55 = 125
125 x .50 + 55 = 117.5 / 118
125 x .60 + 55 = 130
125 x .70 + 55 = 142.5 / 143
125 x .80 + 55 = 155
125 x .90 + 55 = 167.5 / 168

A very basic and typical interval workout might go as follows;

5 minute warm-up @ 50%
4 minutes warm-up @ 60%
1-2 minutes warm-up @ 70%
2 minutes @ 60% (this will be your recovery pace)
2 minutes @ 80% interval
2 minutes @ 60% recovery

2 minutes @ 80% interval
2 minutes @ 60% recovery
2 minutes @ 80% interval
2 minutes @ 60% recovery
2 minutes @ 80% interval

You can hold this pattern of interval (80%) and recovery (60%) for as long as you want. You can even change every other interval to 90%. You can change the times you hold at each interval – it's really up to you and your fitness level. A proper cool down will go something like this;

1-2 minutes cool-down @ 70%
3 minutes cool-down @ 60%
5 minutes cool-down @ 50%

This particular program works out to be 40+/- minutes long but can be expanded and customized to your needs or liking and can be adapted to any exercise, walking, biking, swimming, jogging etc.

The WRAP:

- If you're going to exercise and talk exercise, know what you're talking about.
- Learn about exercise; don't just be "told" what to do, learn the right way and the right meanings of what you're doing.
- Try out the basic interval outline before attempting a Tabata.
- Slow and steady makes you ready.
- Look for Naked Fitness 2 to learn more.

THE FINAL WRAP
(the "naked" ending)

Guys and gals ... this first volume of the Naked Fitness series, was aimed at the absolutely easy and simple idea of getting back to BASICS and just getting started in fitness. If you're already an active exerciser and you picked this up ... sorry if it was too simple, it should be, but hopefully you found one or two nuggets you had forgotten or just didn't know before.

In Naked Fitness 2, I'll be going a lot deeper in the fitness and nutrition sections. You'll be able to know just as much about combining exercises and what body part to work and when, as any trainer out there. In fact the base idea for the second volume is "how to be your own trainer".

In the nutrition section we go a LOT deeper into the whole meal planning, eating and timing, more myth busting about "amped up" foods and drinks ... you'll be able to argue healthy eating how's and whys with the best of them.

The take home message for this entire book is ... just start!! Get to a gym and move your butt as often as possible. Start slow and pick up the pace ONLY when you can and only when it's obvious that you should. If you have some competition aspirations or plans in any sport ... seek out a specialist in that sport and get some ideas on what training you should be doing and if need be ... find yourself a good trainer like we talked about.

Move the body *first* and then deal with the eating. Don't deprive yourself of body fuel and stress out the body at the same time. If you're an experienced exerciser, then this point is mute, you already know what you're doing.

And please ... stay away from the fake "amped-up" foods and pills and drinks that are all over the place. Make a promise to yourself to do this the right way and not cut corners. I promise, you'll feel better and you'll be better off in the long run eating clean and using the best piece of equipment on the planet – your body – to get fit and strong.

It's going to be tough some days and it's going to be easy on others. Learn how to take advantage of both those days and don't stop, don't give up, and don't be talked out of taking care of you!! Make a plan and stick to it. Give yourself a reward for small accomplishments. Stick to your cheat day and EARN your next cheat day.

Good luck ... good fitness ... good eating and good bye for now. I'll see you in Naked Fitness 2!!!

Kevin -